BEST PRACTICES PEDIATRICS

BEST PRACTICES PEDIATRICS

CHARLES RAYMOND BELL, M.D.

Charles Raymond Bell, M.D.

BEST PRACTICES P E D I A T R I C S

Published by Spines

ISBN: 979-8-90222-521-8

Spines

CONTENTS

FOREWORD

Dr. Charles Bell would inevitably author a book that signifies his life's work. You see, he has authored many books on many subjects; however, this one is a sentiment of his lifelong career as a medical doctor. "Best Practices Pediatrics" by Dr. Charles Raymond Bell is a wealth of knowledge for all who read it. There can be multiple uses for this book: How to promote children's health and welfare, ensure safety, provide protocols, and secure parental and community involvement.

I recall the beautiful summer seasons, when our grandmothers sipped lemonade while sitting on the porch. You could hear the melodious sounds of birds, the lavish colors of the flowers in the fields, and the verdant fields promised a lush summer to come. The summer was extremely exciting for we always looked forward to family members coming to visit from nearby states. As children, we were ecstatic to see each other during the summer months.

My attention was always drawn to who I call a favorite cousin, Charles. He was notably smart and talented. He is a songwriter and plays piano in addition to being intelligent and gifted. I admire him and was always inspired by his insightfulness. I always learned something new from him each summer.

As we approached high school, He began to share that he wanted to be a doctor, in fact, a children's doctor. This came as no surprise because I saw him as an achiever, driven by goals and success. He thrived on challenges and loved ticking off accomplishments. Additionally, I found his choice of medical field very suitable. I saw his nurturing characteristics, always focused on caring and supporting others. His strength is empathy and building deep connections. I watched him move on to undergraduate school, then Medical School, residency, and practicing physician.

He immediately began providing medical care to the underserved communities in South Chicago, IL. Later, providing compassionate health care in Pediatrics and Adolescent Medicine in Georgia, Ohio, and Massachusetts, a dedicated career spanning almost four decades. I was so proud to witness his dreams come true through hard work and dedication.

Dr. Charles Bell, a renowned Physician, pediatrician, Health care consultant, and educator, decided to put years of knowledge, hard work, and experience into this book, "Best Practices Pediatrics". I know this book will serve as a conduit and be of value to each student, resident health care practitioner, office administrator, or practicing doctor who wants to have a stellar practice in meeting the needs of Pediatrics. It was a privilege and pleasure to consult with Dr. Bell on this project, especially after having a bird's-eye view since our youth of his love and passion for practicing medicine. As a business professional, I know how critical it is to have the appropriate tools, a reference, or a guideline. This book, "Best Practices Pediatrics", will help conduct day-to-day business and assure everyone who is involved is properly trained in the necessities of how to meet the goals and mission of their medical practice or organization.

Dr. Janice English
Entrepreneur & Educator

INTRODUCTION

In the world of pediatric care, the implementation of best practices holds paramount significance, acting as the cornerstone for the well-being and optimal development of children. This section explores the pivotal role that adherence to established best practices plays in ensuring the delivery of high-quality and compassionate healthcare for the pediatric population, excluding disparities.

One of the primary reasons best practices are crucial in pediatric care is the imperative to ensure the safety of young patients. Children, with their unique physiology and vulnerability, require specialized attention and care. Adhering to evidence-based best practices helps healthcare providers minimize the risks associated with medical interventions and treatments, safeguarding children from potential adverse effects.

By establishing standardized protocols for diagnostics, treatments, and interventions, healthcare professionals can mitigate the likelihood of errors and complications. This not only protects the well-being of the child but also fosters a sense of trust and confidence among parents and caregivers in the healthcare system.

Best practices serve as benchmarks for excellence in pediatric care, guiding healthcare providers toward the most effective and efficient methods of diagnosis, treatment, and ongoing management. These evidence-based guidelines are rooted in the latest research, clinical expertise, and patient outcomes, collectively contributing to an elevated standard of care.

Consistent adherence to best practices promotes the delivery of quality healthcare, thereby improving patient outcomes. Whether it involves routine check-ups, vaccinations, or complex medical interventions, the application of best practices ensures that children receive care that aligns with the latest advancements in the field, fostering positive health trajectories.

Pediatric care often involves multidisciplinary teams, including physicians, nurses, therapists, and other healthcare professionals.

Best practices provide a common framework and language for communication and collaboration among these diverse stakeholders. Standardized guidelines help streamline processes, reduce miscommunication, and enhance the overall coordination of care.

In an era of rapidly evolving medical knowledge, best practices act as a unifying force, ensuring that healthcare providers are on the same page regarding the most effective approaches to pediatric healthcare. This cohesion is especially critical in complex cases that require a comprehensive and integrated approach.

Best practices in pediatric care extend beyond the clinical setting to embrace a holistic, family-centered approach. In recognizing the integral role of parents and caregivers in a child's well-being, these practices encourage open communication, shared decision-making, and the inclusion of family preferences and values in the care plan.

By acknowledging the importance of family dynamics, best practices foster a collaborative partnership between healthcare providers and families. This collaborative model not only enhances the overall quality of care but also empowers families to actively participate in the health and development of their children.

In conclusion, the importance of best practices in pediatric care cannot be overstated. From ensuring safety and minimizing risks to enhancing the quality of care and promoting collaboration, adherence to evidence-based guidelines is essential for the holistic well-being of children and the success of the healthcare system that serves them.

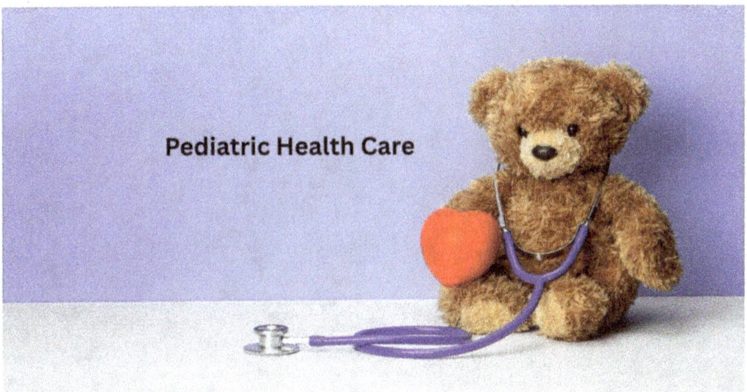

1

A WELCOMING AND SUPPORTIVE ATMOSPHERE

Creating a Welcoming and Supportive Atmosphere for Children and Their Families in Pediatric Best Practices

In the realm of pediatric healthcare, compassion is the cornerstone upon which healing flourishes. Every child deserves to receive care that not only tends to their physical well-being but also nurtures their emotional and psychological needs. This book delves into the essence of compassionate healthcare in pediatrics, offering insights, strategies, and best practices to empower healthcare professionals in providing holistic care to young patients.

The Heart of Pediatric Medicine should always include the fundamental principles of compassionate pediatric care, consisting of empathy, understanding, and patience in building strong relationships with pediatric patients and their families, resulting in a profound impact of compassionate healthcare on children's recovery and overall well-being.

A healing environment goes beyond the physical aspects of a healthcare facility. The significance of creating a welcoming and supportive atmosphere for children and their families may result from colorful and child-friendly spaces to incorporating play and art therapy, with various strategies to promote comfort and alleviate anxiety in pediatric patients.

In pediatric healthcare, the creation of a welcoming and supportive atmosphere for children and their families is a cornerstone of best practices. The pediatric environment profoundly impacts the emotional and psychological well-being of young patients and their caregivers. This chapter explores the importance of fostering such an environment, the elements that contribute to it, and the benefits it brings to both children and their families.

Psychological and Emotional Well-being

Children facing medical treatment often experience anxiety and fear. A welcoming and supportive atmosphere can significantly reduce these negative emotions. By creating a space where children feel safe and cared for, healthcare providers can help mitigate the stress associated with medical visits, leading to a more positive experience.

Trust and Communication

A supportive environment fosters trust between healthcare providers and families. When parents and children feel respected and understood, they are more likely to communicate openly about their concerns and symptoms. This open dialogue is crucial for accurate diagnosis and effective treatment planning.

Enhanced Cooperation and Compliance

Children and families who feel supported are more likely to cooperate with medical procedures and follow treatment plans. When the healthcare environment is perceived as friendly and caring, children are less likely to resist treatments, and parents are more likely to adhere to medical advice, leading to better health outcomes.

Key Elements of a Welcoming and Supportive Atmosphere

Physical Environment

1. **Child-Friendly Design**: Bright, colorful decorations, comfortable furniture, and engaging activities such as toys and books can make the medical setting less intimidating for children.
2. **Safety and Accessibility**: Ensuring that the environment is safe, clean, and easily accessible to all patients, including those with disabilities, is crucial in making everyone feel welcome.

Staff Attitude and Behavior

1. **Empathy and Compassion**: Healthcare providers who demonstrate empathy and compassion can greatly reduce the fear and anxiety of both children and their parents.
2. **Effective Communication**: Using age-appropriate language, being patient, and listening actively to both children and their parents helps build a supportive atmosphere.

Family Involvement

1. **Family-Centered Care:** Involving families in the decision-making process and respecting their knowledge and insights about their child's health fosters a collaborative and supportive environment.
2. **Support Services:** Offering services such as counseling, support groups, and educational

resources can help families feel more supported and empowered in managing their child's health.

Benefits of Welcoming and Supportive Atmosphere

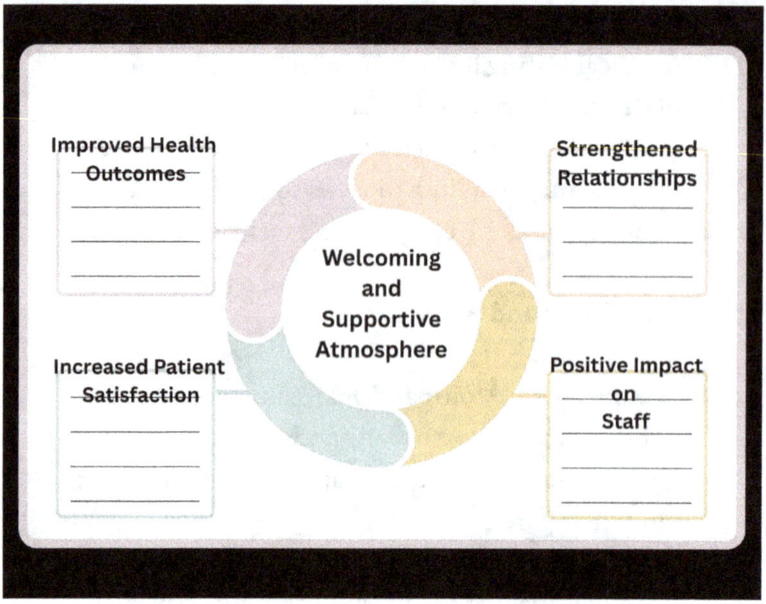

Cultural Sensitivity

1. **Respect for Diversity**: Acknowledging and respecting cultural, religious, and linguistic differences is essential in creating an inclusive and welcoming atmosphere for all families.
2. **Cultural Competence Training**: Providing training for staff on cultural competence can help ensure that all patients and families feel respected and understood.

Benefits of a Welcoming and Supportive Atmosphere

Improved Health Outcomes

Research has shown that children who feel supported and secure are more likely to have better health outcomes. Reduced stress and anxiety can lead to improved immune function, faster recovery times, and a more positive overall experience with the healthcare system.

Increased Patient Satisfaction

Families who feel welcomed and supported are more likely to express satisfaction with the care they receive. High levels of patient satisfaction are linked to better compliance with treatment plans and follow-up appointments, contributing to better long-term health outcomes.

Strengthened Relationships

Building a strong, trust-based relationship between healthcare providers and families enhances the overall quality of care. When families feel connected and valued, they are more likely to remain engaged in their child's healthcare and to seek timely medical advice.

Positive Impact on Staff

A supportive and welcoming atmosphere benefits not only patients and families but also healthcare providers. Staff members who work in a positive environment are more likely to experience job satisfaction, reduced burnout, and a stronger commitment to providing high-quality care.

CONCLUSION

Creating a welcoming and supportive atmosphere for children and their families is an integral part of pediatric best practices. By focusing on the physical environment, staff attitudes, family involvement, and cultural sensitivity, healthcare providers can significantly enhance the quality of care they offer. The benefits of such an approach are far-reaching, leading to improved health outcomes, higher patient satisfaction, and stronger, more trusting relationships between families and healthcare providers. Investing in a supportive and welcoming atmosphere is not only beneficial for patients and their families but also for the healthcare system as a whole, promoting a more compassionate and effective approach to pediatric care.

CLEAR AND COMPASSIONATE COMMUNICATION IN PEDIATRIC HEALTHCARE

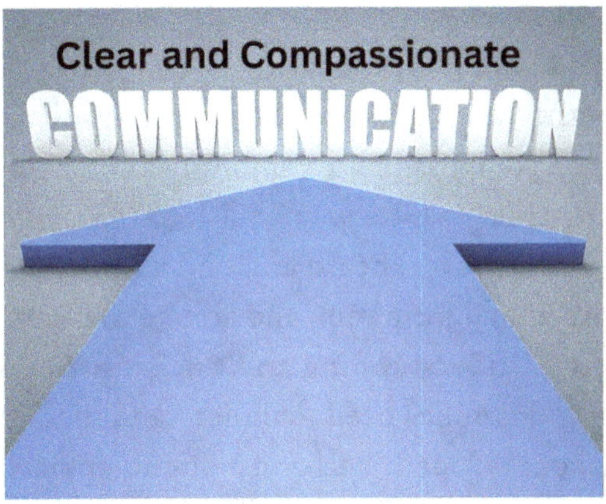

Effective communication is paramount in pediatric healthcare. Emphasis must be placed on the importance of clear and compassionate communication between healthcare professionals, patients, and their families for the communication to be effective. Techniques for conveying complex medical information in a manner that is age-appropriate, understandable, and respectful of cultural differences are very important.

Furthermore, the benefits of collaboration among multidisciplinary teams in delivering comprehensive care should be focused upon and planned as achievable goals.

Effective communication in healthcare is essential for delivering high-quality care, particularly in pediatrics, where the needs and understanding of patients and their families vary widely. Clear and compassionate communication between healthcare professionals, patients, and their families fosters trust, ensures accurate information transfer, and promotes better health outcomes. This section delves into the importance of such communication, techniques for conveying complex medical information in an understandable and culturally sensitive manner, and the benefits of collaboration among multidisciplinary teams in providing comprehensive care.

Building Trust and Rapport

Trust is the foundation of the patient-provider relationship. Clear and compassionate communication helps build and maintain this trust, which is crucial for effective care. When patients and families feel heard and understood, they are more likely to share vital information and adhere to treatment plans.

Enhancing Understanding and Decision-Making

Patients and families need to understand medical information to make informed decisions about their care. Clear communication ensures they grasp the nature of their condition, treatment options, and potential outcomes, empowering them to participate actively in their healthcare journey.

Reducing Anxiety and Fear

Medical environments can be intimidating, especially for children and their families. Compassionate communication can alleviate anxiety and fear, making the experience less daunting and more supportive.

Ensuring Adherence to Treatment Plans

When patients and families understand the reasons behind treatment recommendations and feel confident in the care they are receiving, they are more likely to follow through with prescribed treatments and attend follow-up appointments. As healthcare providers, let's help our patients and their parents say "NO" to no-shows.

Techniques for Conveying Complex Medical Information

Age-Appropriate Communication

1. **Simplified Language**: Use simple, straightforward language when explaining medical terms. Avoid jargon and technical terms unless they are clearly defined.
2. **Visual Aids**: Diagrams, models, and videos can help illustrate complex concepts in a way that is easier for children to understand. If financially possible, educational videos can be effectively placed in waiting room areas while patients are waiting for appointments.
3. **Interactive Methods**: Engage children with questions and activities that help them learn about their condition and treatment interactively and memorably.

Cultural Sensitivity

1. **Cultural Competence**: Understand and respect cultural differences that may influence how patients and families perceive health, illness, and medical care.

2. **Language Services**: Provide translation and interpretation services to ensure that non-English-speaking families receive accurate and comprehensible information. Use certified interpreters versus non-certified interpreters.
3. **Culturally Relevant Examples**: Use examples and analogies that are culturally relevant to help explain medical concepts in a way that resonates with the patient's background and experiences.

Respectful Communication

1. **Active Listening**: Show that you are listening by nodding, making eye contact, and responding appropriately. It is important to validate the patient’s and family's feelings and concerns.
2. **Empathy and Compassion**: Express empathy and understanding. Acknowledge the emotional and psychological impact of the medical condition on the patient and their family.

3. **Respecting Autonomy**: Involve patients and families in the decision-making process, respecting their right to make choices about their care.

Collaboration Among Multidisciplinary Teams

Comprehensive Care

1. **Holistic Approach**: Multidisciplinary teams bring together diverse expertise to address all aspects of a patient's health, including physical, emotional, and social needs.

2. **Coordinated Care**: Effective communication and collaboration among team members ensure that care is well-coordinated, reducing the risk of fragmented or contradictory treatment plans.

Improved Outcomes

1. **Shared Knowledge**: Team members share their knowledge and expertise, leading to more accurate diagnoses and more effective treatment plans.
2. **Enhanced Problem-Solving**: Diverse perspectives within a multidisciplinary team can lead to innovative solutions to complex medical issues.

Patient and Family Support

1. **Comprehensive Support**: Teams that include social workers, psychologists, and other support staff can provide comprehensive support to patients and families, addressing not only medical but also emotional and social needs.
2. **Continuity of Care**: Multidisciplinary teams can ensure continuity of care, with each team member contributing to a cohesive care plan that follows the patient through different stages of treatment.

Benefits of Clear and Compassionate Communication and Multidisciplinary Collaboration

Patient Satisfaction

Patients and families who experience clear, compassionate communication and coordinated care from a multidisciplinary team report higher levels of satisfaction. They feel more supported, respected, and confident in the care they receive.

Better Health Outcomes

Clear communication and effective multidisciplinary collaboration lead to better health outcomes. Patients receive comprehensive, coordinated care, reducing the likelihood of medical errors, improving adherence to treatment plans, and promoting faster recovery.

Enhanced Team Efficiency

When healthcare professionals communicate effectively and work collaboratively, the efficiency and effectiveness of the healthcare team are enhanced. This leads to better resource utilization, reduced duplication of efforts, and a more streamlined care process.

Professional Satisfaction

Healthcare providers who engage in clear, compassionate communication and effective collaboration with their colleagues experience higher job satisfaction. They feel more connected to their patients, their colleagues, and their work, leading to a more positive work environment.

CONCLUSION

Clear and compassionate communication between healthcare professionals, patients, and their families is vital for effective pediatric care. It builds trust, enhances understanding, reduces anxiety, and ensures adherence to treatment plans. Employing techniques for conveying complex medical information in an age-appropriate, understandable, and culturally respectful manner further supports these goals.

Additionally, collaboration among multidisciplinary teams provides comprehensive, coordinated care that addresses the holistic needs of patients and families.

Together, these practices lead to improved health

outcomes, higher patient and professional satisfaction, and a more efficient and effective healthcare system. Investing in communication skills and fostering a collaborative environment is essential for delivering the highest standard of pediatric care.

STRATEGIES TO ADDRESS EMOTIONAL NEEDS

Strategies to Address Emotional Needs for Pediatric Patients of All Ages

EMOTIONAL NEEDS OF CHILDREN

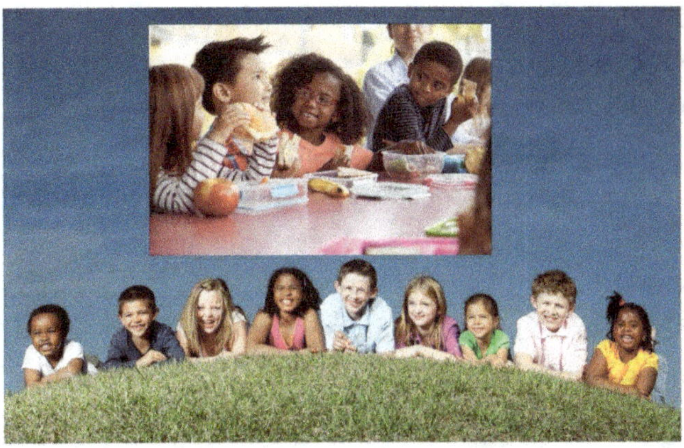

Introduction

Pediatric patients often experience a wide range of emotions when undergoing medical treatment. Addressing these emotional needs with sensitivity and compassion is crucial for providing holistic care that supports not only the physical but also the emotional well-being of children. This section explores strategies to address the emotional needs of pediatric patients across different age groups, emphasizing the importance of tailoring approaches to the unique developmental and individual needs of each child.

Understanding Emotional Needs in Pediatric Patients

Infants (0-2 years)

Infants primarily communicate through crying, facial expressions, and body language. Their emotional needs are closely tied to their physical comfort and security.

Toddlers (2-4 years)

Toddlers begin to express themselves verbally but still rely heavily on caregivers for emotional support. They may experience fear and anxiety in unfamiliar environments.

Preschoolers (4-6 years)

Preschoolers have more advanced language skills and can express their emotions more clearly. They may have specific fears about medical procedures and a vivid imagination that can amplify their anxieties.

School-age Children (6-12 years)

School-age children understand more complex concepts and can communicate their thoughts and feelings effectively. They may worry about the impact of their illness on their daily activities and social interactions.

Adolescents (12-18 years)

Adolescents are capable of abstract thinking and have a strong desire for independence. They may experience a range of emotions, including anger, frustration, and concern about their future.

Strategies for Addressing Emotional Needs

Creating a Safe and Supportive Environment

1. **Comfortable Setting**: Ensure the physical environment is child-friendly, with bright colors, toys, and decorations that make the space less intimidating.
2. **Consistent Routine**: Maintain a consistent routine to help children feel secure and understand what to expect during their visit.

Building Trust and Rapport

1. **Introduce Yourself**: Always introduce yourself and explain your role to the child and their family.
2. **Eye Level Communication**: Get down to the child's eye level to make communication feel more personal and less intimidating.
3. **Active Listening**: Listen attentively to the child's concerns and validate their feelings.

Tailoring Communication to Developmental Levels

1. **Use Simple Language**: Use age-appropriate language and avoid medical jargon when explaining procedures or treatments.
2. **Visual Aids and Demonstrations**: Use pictures, models, and demonstrations to help explain what will happen during medical procedures.

3. **Storytelling and Play**: Use storytelling and play to help younger children understand and cope with their experiences.

Providing Emotional Support

1. **Reassurance and Encouragement**: Offer frequent reassurance and encouragement, acknowledging the child's bravery and cooperation.
2. **Comfort Items**: Allow children to bring comfort items, such as a favorite toy or blanket, to medical appointments and procedures.
3. **Parental Involvement**: Encourage parents to be present and involved in their child's care, providing emotional support and comfort.

Addressing Specific Fears and Anxieties

1. **Pre-Procedure Preparation**: Explain procedures in advance, using age-appropriate language and tools. Allow the child to ask questions and express their fears.
2. **Coping Techniques**: Teach and practice coping techniques such as deep breathing, visualization, or progressive muscle relaxation.
3. **Distraction Methods**: Use distraction methods such as videos, games, or music during medical procedures to help reduce anxiety.

Encouraging Expression of Emotions

1. **Open Dialogue**: Create an environment where

children feel safe to express their emotions and ask questions.

2. **Art and Play Therapy**: Use art and play therapy to help children express their feelings and work through their anxieties in a non-verbal way.
3. **Journaling and Writing**: Encourage older children and adolescents to journal or write about their experiences and feelings.

Providing Support for Parents and Caregivers

1. **Educational Resources**: Provide parents with educational resources to help them understand their child's emotional needs and how to support them.
2. **Counseling and Support Groups**: Offer counseling services and support groups for parents to help them cope with the emotional challenges of caring for a sick child.
3. **Encourage Self-Care**: Remind parents to take care of their own emotional and physical well-being so they can be a stable support system for their child.

Multidisciplinary Approach

1. **Collaboration with Specialists**: Collaborate with child psychologists, social workers, and other specialists to address the emotional needs of pediatric patients comprehensively.
2. **Integrated Care Plans**: Develop integrated care plans that include strategies for addressing both the physical and emotional needs of the child. The

> most important benefit of integrated health is the improved results patients experience.[14]

Benefits of Addressing Emotional Needs with Sensitivity and Compassion

Improved Patient Outcomes

Addressing emotional needs can lead to better compliance with treatment, reduced anxiety and stress, and overall improved health outcomes for pediatric patients.

Enhanced Patient and Family Satisfaction

When children and their families feel supported emotionally, they are more likely to have a positive experience with the healthcare system and express higher levels of satisfaction with their care.

Stronger Patient-Provider Relationships

Compassionate and sensitive care fosters trust and strengthens the relationship between healthcare providers and families, leading to more effective communication and collaboration.

Reduced Healthcare Costs

By addressing emotional needs and reducing anxiety, healthcareproviders can potentially reduce the need for sedation, lower the incidence of complications, and decrease the length of hospital stays.

Conclusion

Addressing the emotional needs of pediatric patients with sensitivity and compassion is essential for providing comprehensive and effective healthcare. By creating a safe and supportive environment, building trust, tailoring communication to developmental levels, and involving families, healthcare providers can significantly enhance the emotional well-being of their young patients. Implementing these strategies not only improves health outcomes but also fosters positive experiences and strong relationships between patients, families, and healthcare providers.

FAMILY-CENTERED CARE/FOSTERING RESILIENCE

FAMILY-CENTERED CARE AND FOSTERING RESILIENCE IN PEDIATRIC HEALTHCARE

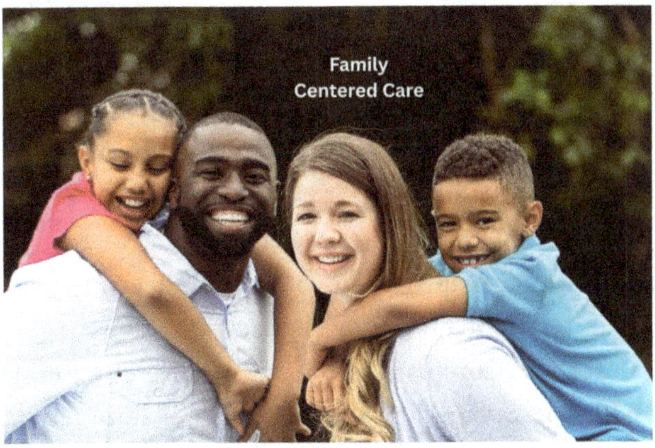

Family-centered care is an approach that recognizes the vital role families play in the health and well-being of pediatric patients. It involves collaborating with families to provide care that respects their needs, values, and preferences. An essential aspect of family-centered care is fostering resilience in children and their families, helping them navigate and overcome the challenges posed by health issues. This section explores the principles of family-centered care, the importance of fostering resilience, and the strategies healthcare professionals can use to support families through resilience-building interventions, coping strategies, and support networks.

Family-Centered Care

Principles of Family-Centered Care

1. **Respect and Dignity**: Healthcare providers listen to and honor the perspectives and choices of patients and their families. Families' knowledge, values, beliefs, and cultural backgrounds are incorporated into the planning and delivery of care.
2. **Information Sharing**: Providers communicate and share complete, unbiased information with families in ways that are affirming and useful. Families receive timely, complete, and accurate information to effectively participate in care and decision-making.
3. **Participation**: Families are encouraged and supported to participate in care and decision-making at the level they choose.
4. **Collaboration**: Patients, families, and providers collaborate in policy and program development, implementation, and evaluation, as well as in the delivery of care.

Benefits of Family-Centered Care

1. **Enhanced Patient and Family Satisfaction**: Families feel respected and valued, leading to higher satisfaction with the healthcare experience.
2. **Improved Health Outcomes**: Involving families in care leads to better adherence to treatment plans, reduced anxiety, and improved health outcomes for children.
3. **Stronger Family-Provider Relationships**: Collaboration and open communication foster trust and strengthen relationships between families and healthcare providers.

Fostering Resilience in the Face of Adversity

Understanding Resilience

Resilience is the ability to adapt and recover from adversity, stress, or trauma. It involves a combination of internal strengths and external resources that help individuals and families cope with challenges and bounce back stronger.

Importance of Resilience in Pediatric Healthcare

1. **Coping with Medical Challenges**: Resilience helps children and families manage the emotional and psychological stress associated with illness, treatment, and hospitalization.
2. **Long-Term Well-Being**: Building resilience contributes to long-term mental and emotional well-being, helping individuals maintain a positive outlook despite ongoing health challenges.
3. **Empowerment and Confidence**: Resilient families feel more empowered and confident in their ability to handle future challenges, leading to better overall health management.

Strategies for Building Resilience

Resilience-Building Interventions

1. **Positive Reinforcement and Encouragement**: Provide positive feedback and encouragement to help children and families recognize their strengths and achievements.
2. **Skill-Building Activities**: Engage children in activities that build problem-solving skills, self-efficacy, and emotional regulation.
3. **Therapeutic Interventions**: Utilize therapies such as cognitive-behavioral therapy (CBT) and play therapy to help children develop coping strategies and resilience.

Coping Strategies

1. **Stress Management Techniques**: Teach children and families stress management techniques such as deep breathing, mindfulness, and relaxation exercises.
2. **Healthy Routines**: Encourage the establishment of healthy routines, including regular sleep, nutritious meals, and physical activity, to promote overall well-being.
3. **Goal Setting**: Help families set realistic and achievable goals, providing a sense of purpose and direction during challenging times.

Support Networks

1. **Peer Support Groups**: Facilitate peer support groups where families can share experiences, offer mutual support, and learn from each other's coping strategies.
2. **Community Resources**: Connect families with community resources, such as counseling services, financial assistance programs, and educational workshops.
3. **Family Support Services**: Provide access to family support services, including social work, chaplaincy, and behavioral health services, to address the diverse needs of families.

The Role of Healthcare Professionals

Creating a Supportive Environment

1. **Empathy and Compassion**: Show empathy and compassion in all interactions, recognizing the emotional and psychological impact of health challenges on children and families.
2. **Safe Space for Expression**: Create a safe space where children and families feel comfortable expressing their fears, concerns, and emotions.

Educating and Empowering Families

1. **Educational Resources**: Provide families with educational resources about their child's condition, treatment options, and coping strategies.
2. **Empowerment Through Knowledge**: Empower families by involving them in care decisions and encouraging them to ask questions and seek information.

Collaboration and Coordination of Care

1. **Multidisciplinary Teams**: Collaborate with multidisciplinary teams, including doctors, nurses, social workers, and therapists, to provide comprehensive and coordinated care.
2. **Continuity of Care**: Ensure continuity of care by maintaining open communication and collaboration among all members of the healthcare team.

ROLE OF HEALTHCARE PROFESSIONALS

CONCLUSION

Family-centered care and resilience-building are integral components of pediatric healthcare. By respecting and involving families, healthcare professionals can create a supportive environment that fosters trust, enhances patient satisfaction, and improves health outcomes. Building resilience in children and their families through targeted interventions, effective coping strategies, and strong support networks empowers them to navigate the challenges of illness and emerge stronger. Investing in these approaches not only benefits individual patients and families but also strengthens the overall healthcare system, promoting a more compassionate and effective model of care.

2

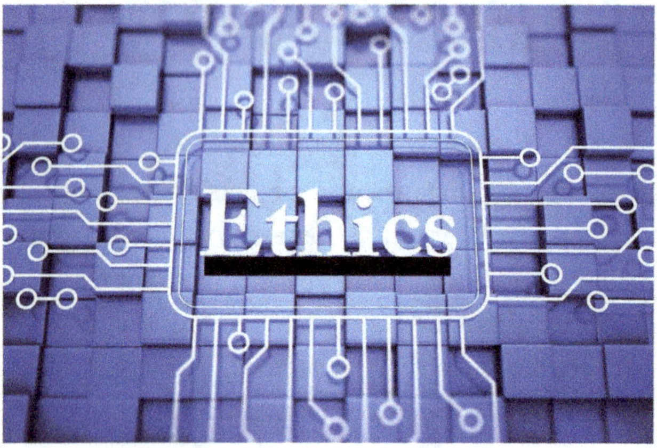

ETHICAL CONSIDERATIONS

ETHICAL CONSIDERATIONS IN PEDIATRIC HEALTHCARE

Introduction

Ethical considerations in pediatric healthcare are complex and multifaceted, involving the delicate balance between the rights and best interests of the child, the role of the family, and the responsibilities of healthcare professionals. Key issues include informed consent, privacy, and end-of-life care. Healthcare professionals frequently encounter ethical dilemmas and must navigate these challenges with compassion and integrity. This chapter explores these ethical issues and provides guidance on addressing them in a manner that upholds ethical principles and supports the well-being of pediatric patients and their families.

Informed Consent in Pediatric Healthcare

The Concept of Informed Consent

Informed consent is the process by which patients or their legal guardians receive comprehensive information about a medical procedure or treatment, understand its risks and benefits, and voluntarily agree to it. In pediatric healthcare, obtaining informed consent involves both parents or guardians and, when appropriate, the child.

Challenges in Pediatric Informed Consent

1 Capacity and Comprehension: Children's ability to understand medical information varies with age and developmental stage. Assessing their capacity to comprehend and participate in the decision-making process is crucial.

2 Parental Authority and Child Assent: Parents or guardians generally provide consent for minors, but involving the child and obtaining their assent respects their developing autonomy and encourages their participation in their care.

3 Conflict of Interests: Situations may arise where parents' decisions may not align with what healthcare providers believe to be in the child's best interests, leading to ethical dilemmas.

Best Practices for Informed Consent

1 Developmentally Appropriate Communication: Tailor explanations to the child's developmental level, using language and concepts they can understand.

2 Shared Decision-Making: Involve the child in the decision-making process as much as possible, respecting their growing autonomy and encouraging their input.

3 Clear and Transparent Communication: Ensure that parents or guardians receive clear, complete, and unbiased information about the proposed treatments, risks, benefits, and alternatives.

Privacy and Confidentiality

Importance of Privacy and Confidentiality

Privacy and confidentiality are fundamental rights in

healthcare, ensuring that personal and medical information is protected. In pediatrics, safeguarding these rights is essential to maintain trust between patients, families, and healthcare providers.

Challenges in Pediatric Privacy

1 Parental Access to Information: Balancing the child's right to privacy with parents' need for information can be challenging, especially as children approach adolescence.

2 Confidentiality in Sensitive Issues: Issues such as sexual health, behavioral health, and substance use may require special consideration to respect the child's privacy and confidentiality.

3 Electronic Health Records: The increasing use of electronic health records (EHRs) presents challenges in maintaining confidentiality, as information may be more easily accessed or shared.

ENSURING PRIVACY AND CONFIDENTIALITY

Best Practices for Ensuring Privacy and Confidentiality

1 Age-Appropriate Confidentiality: Gradually increase the level of confidentiality provided to the child as they mature, respecting their evolving capacity for privacy.

2 Clear Policies and Communication: Develop and communicate clear policies regarding confidentiality to both children and their families, explaining how information will be protected and shared.

3 Secure Information Systems: Implement robust security measures for EHRs to protect patient information from unauthorized access or breaches.

End-of-Life Care

Ethical Considerations in Pediatric End-of-Life Care

End-of-life care in pediatrics involves unique ethical challenges, as decisions must balance the best interests of the child, the wishes of the family, and the professional responsibilities of healthcare providers.

1 Best Interests of the Child: Determining what constitutes the best interests of the child can be complex, involving considerations of quality of life, potential suffering, and the child's expressed wishes.

2 Parental Decision-Making: Parents or guardians often face profound emotional challenges in making end-of-life decisions for their children, and their perspectives must be sensitively navigated.

3 Palliative Care: Integrating palliative care principles, including pain management, emotional support, and quality of life considerations, is essential in end-of-life care.

Best Practices for End-of-Life Care

1 Comprehensive Communication: Maintain open, honest, and compassionate communication with families, providing clear information and supporting them through difficult decisions.

2 Multidisciplinary Approach: Utilize a multidisciplinary team to provide comprehensive care, including medical, psychological, and spiritual support for the child and their family.

3 Respect for Autonomy: When possible, involve the child in discussions about their care and respect their preferences and values, balancing this with parental input and professional judgment.

Navigating Ethical Dilemmas

Common Ethical Dilemmas in Pediatric Healthcare

1 Refusal of Treatment: Parents may refuse recommended treatments for their child, leading to conflicts between respecting parental authority and ensuring the child's best interests.

2 Resource Allocation: Decisions about the allocation of limited resources, such as organ transplants or experimental treatments, can present ethical challenges.

3 Cultural and Religious Beliefs: Differences in cultural and religious beliefs about medical care can lead to ethical dilemmas and require sensitive negotiation.

Strategies for Navigating Ethical Dilemmas

1 **Ethics Consultations**: Seek input from ethics committees or consultants to help resolve complex ethical issues and provide balanced, well-considered guidance.

2 **Interdisciplinary Collaboration**: Work collaboratively with an interdisciplinary team, including medical, legal, social work, and ethical experts, to address ethical dilemmas from multiple perspectives.

3 **Continuous Education**: Engage in ongoing education about ethical principles and dilemmas in pediatric healthcare to enhance knowledge and preparedness for ethical challenges.

Conclusion

Ethical considerations in pediatric healthcare require careful attention to informed consent, privacy, and end-of-life care, among other issues. Healthcare professionals must navigate these challenges with compassion and integrity, ensuring that the best interests of the child are always prioritized while respecting the roles and rights of families. By employing best practices in communication, decision-making, and multidisciplinary collaboration, healthcare providers can uphold ethical principles and support the well-being of pediatric patients and their families.

Continuous Improvement

In the pursuit of excellence in pediatric healthcare, continuous improvement is essential. Compassionate healthcare in pediatrics is not merely a practice but a philosophy—a commitment to nurturing the young lives entrusted to our care. By embracing empathy, fostering resilience, and prioritizing the holistic well-being of pediatric patients and their families, we can create a brighter and healthier future for generations to come.

In this book, the goal is to provide healthcare professionals with a comprehensive guide to integrating compassion into every aspect of pediatric care, ultimately transforming the healthcare experience for children and their families.

FOUNDATIONAL CONCEPTS OF SAFETY

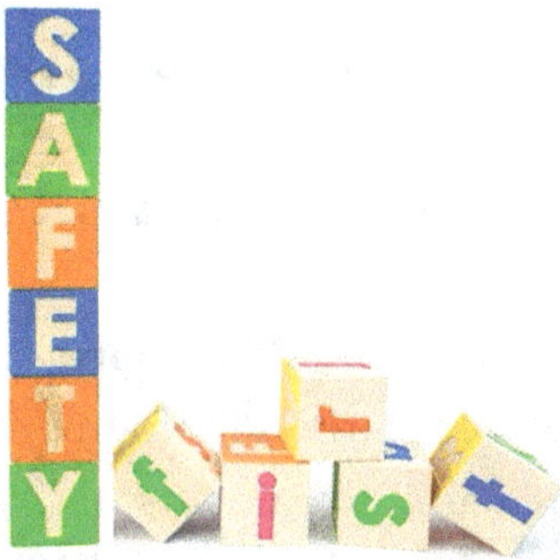

FOUNDATIONAL CONCEPTS OF SAFETY IN PEDIATRIC HEALTHCARE

Safe Haven: Ensuring Pediatric Healthcare Excellence through Safety Protocols

Safety is paramount in pediatric healthcare. Every child deserves to receive care in an environment that prioritizes their well-being and minimizes the risk of harm. This section serves as a comprehensive guide to safety protocols and best practices in pediatric healthcare, empowering healthcare professionals to create safe and secure environments for young patients.

Safety in pediatric healthcare is paramount due to the unique vulnerabilities of pediatric patients. Ensuring the safety of children in healthcare settings involves protecting their physical, emotional, and psychological well-being. Implementing robust safety protocols and strategies for preventing medical errors is essential to mitigate risks and promote a culture of safety. This section explores foundational safety concepts, the specific vulnerabilities of pediatric patients, and effective strategies for preventing medical errors, including medication safety, infection control, and patient identification protocols.

Foundational Concepts of Safety in Pediatric Healthcare

Unique Vulnerabilities of Pediatric Patients

1. **Developmental Considerations**: Children's physical and cognitive development stages can impact their ability to understand and communicate their health needs.
2. **Physiological Differences**: Pediatric patients have different physiological responses to medications and treatments compared to adults, necessitating age-specific dosages and approaches.
3. **Dependency on Caregivers**: Children depend heavily on caregivers for their care, making it crucial to involve and educate families in safety practices.
4. **Emotional and Psychological Impact**: Hospitalization and medical procedures can be

particularly stressful for children, affecting their emotional and psychological well-being.

Importance of Robust Safety Protocols

1. **Preventing Harm**: Safety protocols help prevent physical harm, medical errors, and adverse events, ensuring a secure environment for pediatric patients.
2. **Promoting Trust**: Ensuring safety builds trust between healthcare providers, patients, and families, essential for effective healthcare delivery.
3. **Improving Outcomes**: Implementing safety measures contributes to better health outcomes and overall patient satisfaction.

Strategies for Preventing Medical Errors

Medication Safety

1. **Weight-Based Dosing**: Use weight-based dosing calculations to ensure accurate medication dosages for pediatric patients.
2. **Double-Check Systems**: Implement double-check systems for high-risk medications, involving two healthcare professionals in the verification process.
3. **Standardized Protocols**: Develop and adhere to standardized protocols for prescribing, dispensing, and administering medications.
4. **Patient and Family Education**: Educate patients and families about medication administration, potential side effects, and the importance of adhering to prescribed regimens.

Infection Control

1. **Hand Hygiene**: Emphasize the importance of hand hygiene among healthcare providers, patients, and families to prevent the spread of infections.
2. **Vaccination**: Ensure that all healthcare personnel are up to date with vaccinations to protect against communicable diseases.
3. **Sterilization and Disinfection**: Follow strict sterilization and disinfection protocols for medical equipment and patient care areas.
4. **Isolation Precautions**: Implement appropriate isolation precautions for patients with contagious diseases to prevent cross-infection.

BEST PRACTICES FOR MITIGATING RISKS

Patient Identification Protocols

1. **Accurate Identification**: Use multiple identifiers (e.g., name, date of birth) to verify patient identity before administering treatments or procedures.
2. **Barcode Systems**: Implement barcode scanning systems for patient identification and medication administration to reduce errors.
3. **Clear Communication**: Ensure clear and effective communication among healthcare team members regarding patient identification and care plans.
4. **Education and Training**: Provide ongoing education and training for healthcare providers on the importance of accurate patient identification and the protocols to follow.

Best Practices for Mitigating Risks and Promoting Patient Safety

Creating a Culture of Safety

1. **Leadership Commitment**: Ensure that healthcare leadership is committed to promoting a culture of safety, emphasizing the importance of safety at all organizational levels.
2. **Safety Reporting Systems**: Implement non-punitive reporting systems for safety concerns and near-misses to encourage reporting and learning from incidents.
3. **Regular Training and Education**: Provide regular training and continuing education for healthcare providers on safety protocols, error prevention, and best practices.

Implementing Safety Protocols

1. **Checklists and Protocols**: Utilize checklists and standardized protocols to guide clinical practice and reduce variability in care.
2. **Technology and Innovation**: Leverage technology, such as electronic health records (EHRs) and computerized physician order entry (CPOE) systems, to enhance accuracy and reduce errors.
3. **Team-Based Care**: Promote team-based care approaches that emphasize collaboration, communication, and shared responsibility for patient safety.

Patient and Family Engagement

1. **Education and Involvement**: Educate patients and families about safety practices and involve them in care decisions to enhance their understanding and adherence to safety measures.

2. **Feedback Mechanisms**: Establish feedback mechanisms for patients and families to share safety concerns and suggestions for improvement.

Continuous Improvement

1. **Root Cause Analysis**: Conduct root cause analyses of adverse events and near-misses to identify underlying issues and implement corrective actions.
2. **Quality Improvement Initiatives**: Engage in continuous quality improvement initiatives that focus on identifying, implementing, and evaluating interventions to enhance patient safety.
3. **Ensuring Facility Safety**

Creation of a safe environment requires focusing on ensuring facility safety as being just as important as other safety protocols for providing safe and quality healthcare for pediatric patients.

3

CREATING A SAFE ENVIRONMENT IN PEDIATRIC HEALTHCARE FACILITIES

Creating a safe environment in pediatric healthcare extends beyond clinical practices to include the physical infrastructure of healthcare facilities. This encompasses building design, equipment maintenance, and emergency preparedness plans. Prioritizing facility safety is essential for minimizing hazards and ensuring a secure environment for pediatric patients, their families, and healthcare staff. This chapter explores the key aspects of creating a safe physical environment in pediatric healthcare settings and provides strategies for implementing best practices.

Building Design for Safety

Child-Friendly and Safe Design

1. Age-Appropriate Spaces: Design spaces that cater to different age groups with appropriate furniture, toys, and activities to reduce anxiety and create a welcoming atmosphere.

2. Safe Play Areas: Include designated play areas that are safe and visible to parents and staff, minimizing the risk of accidents.

Infection Control Through Design

1. Separate Waiting Areas: Design separate waiting areas for sick and well children to reduce the risk of cross-infection.
2. Hand Hygiene Stations: Install hand hygiene stations at key locations, such as entrances, exam rooms, and near restrooms, to encourage frequent handwashing.

Accessibility and Mobility

1. Universal Design: Ensure that the facility is accessible to children with disabilities, including ramps, elevators, and appropriately sized doorways.
2. Wayfinding: Implement clear and simple signage to help families navigate the facility easily and reduce stress.

Safety Features

1. Non-Slip Flooring: Use non-slip flooring materials to prevent falls, especially in areas prone to spills such as bathrooms and cafeterias.
2. Secure Windows and Doors: Install childproof locks on windows and doors to prevent accidents and unauthorized access.

Equipment Maintenance

Regular Inspection and Maintenance

1. Routine Checks: Implement a schedule for regular inspection and maintenance of medical and non-medical equipment to ensure functionality and safety.
2. Prompt Repairs: Establish protocols for promptly addressing and repairing any equipment malfunctions or damages to prevent accidents.

Training and Competency

1. Staff Training: Provide comprehensive training for staff on the proper use and maintenance of equipment to minimize errors and accidents.
2. Competency Assessments: Conduct regular competency assessments to ensure that staff are proficient in using and maintaining equipment safely.

Emergency Preparedness

Comprehensive Emergency Plans

1. Emergency Response Plans: Develop and regularly update comprehensive emergency response plans covering various scenarios such as fires, natural disasters, and medical emergencies.
2. Evacuation Routes: Clearly mark and regularly practice evacuation routes to ensure all staff and families are familiar with the procedures.

Regular Drills and Training

1. Emergency Drills: Conduct regular emergency drills to test the effectiveness of response plans and identify areas for improvement.
2. Staff Training: Provide ongoing training for staff on emergency procedures, including the use of emergency equipment and first aid.

Creating a Culture of Safety
Leadership Commitment

1. Safety as a Priority: Ensure that safety is a top priority for the organization, with visible commitment from leadership to support safety initiatives.
2. Open Communication: Foster an environment where staff feel comfortable reporting safety concerns and near-misses without fear of retribution.

Continuous Improvement

1. Regular Audits: Conduct regular safety audits to identify potential hazards and areas for improvement (i.e., twice a year).
2. Feedback Mechanisms: Implement systems for collecting and acting on feedback from staff, patients, and families to continuously enhance safety measures.

Examples of Implementation of Protocols:

1: Designing a Child-Friendly Pediatric Ward

A pediatric hospital designs its new ward with input from child development experts and families. The result is a vibrant, child-friendly environment with age-appropriate play areas, non-slip flooring, and secure windows. This design not only improves safety but also enhances the overall experience for children and families.

2: Effective Equipment Maintenance Program

A community health center implements a robust equipment maintenance program, including regular inspections and prompt repairs. Staff receive ongoing training on equipment use and safety. This proactive approach reduces equipment-related accidents and ensures reliable care.

3: Successful Emergency Preparedness Drill

A pediatric clinic conducts a comprehensive fire drill, involving staff, patients, and families. The drill identifies several areas for improvement, including clearer signage and more frequent training. After addressing these issues, the clinic reports increased confidence in its emergency response capabilities.

Conclusion

Creating a safe environment in pediatric healthcare facilities requires a comprehensive approach that extends beyond clinical practices. By focusing on building design, equipment maintenance, and emergency preparedness, healthcare organizations can minimize hazards and create a secure environment for pediatric patients, families, and staff. Prioritizing facility safety not only prevents accidents and emergencies but also fosters a culture of safety and trust, ultimately enhancing the quality of care provided. Through continuous improvement and a commitment to safety, healthcare facilities can ensure a safe and welcoming environment for all. By fostering a culture of safety, engaging patients and families, and committing to continuous improvement, healthcare providers can protect the physical, emotional, and psychological well-being of children and ensure a safe and supportive healthcare environment.

GENERAL SAFETY IN PEDIATRIC HEALTHCARE-BEST PRACTICES

Safe Medication Practices and Infection Prevention

Ensuring the safety and well-being of pediatric patients requires meticulous attention to medication practices, infection prevention, and safe patient transport. This section outlines best practices for prescribing, administering, and monitoring medications in pediatric patients, highlights the importance of preventing healthcare-associated infections, and discusses strategies for safe patient transport.

Safe Medication Practices

Best Practices for Prescribing Medications

1. **Accurate Dosage Calculations**: Pediatric dosages must be calculated based on weight or body surface area to avoid underdosing or overdosing. Always double-check calculations and use standardized dosing tools.
2. **Age-Appropriate Formulations**: Select medications that are suitable for the child's age,

considering liquid formulations for young children who cannot swallow pills.

3. **Comprehensive Medication History**: Gather a complete medication history, including over-the-counter drugs, supplements, and any allergies, to prevent adverse drug interactions. Appropriately reconcile the list of medications at each visit.

Administering Medications

1. **Double-Check System**: Implement a double-check system where two healthcare professionals verify the medication, dosage, and patient identity before administration. Check for the expiration date before administering medication.
2. **Parental Involvement**: Educate parents about the medications their child is receiving, including the purpose, dosage, and potential side effects. Involve them in the administration process when appropriate. Warn the parents or guardians against increasing or decreasing dosages without the provider's permission.
3. **Child-Friendly Techniques**: Use distraction techniques, such as storytelling or toys, to ease the child's anxiety during medication administration.

Monitoring and Reconciliation by Providers

1. **Regular Monitoring**: Monitor the child for any adverse reactions or side effects following medication administration. Adjust dosages as needed based on response and side effects.

2. **Medication Reconciliation**: Perform thorough medication reconciliation when hospitalized, at every transition of care (e.g., admission, transfer, discharge) or during each office visit to ensure accuracy and continuity in medication management.

Reducing Medication Errors

1. **Electronic Prescribing Systems**: Use electronic prescribing systems with built-in safety checks to reduce errors related to handwriting, dosage calculations, and drug interactions.
2. **Standardized Protocols**: Develop and adhere to standardized protocols for high-risk medications and processes, such as chemotherapy and anesthesia.
3. **Continuous Education**: Provide ongoing education and training for healthcare professionals on safe medication practices and error-prevention strategies.

Preventing Healthcare-Associated Infections (HAIs)
Importance of Infection Prevention and Control

1. **Vulnerable Populations**: Pediatric patients, especially neonates and immunocompromised children, are highly susceptible to infections. Preventing HAIs is critical to protecting these vulnerable populations.
2. **Reducing Morbidity and Mortality**: Effective infection prevention measures reduce the incidence

of HAIs, which in turn decreases morbidity, mortality, and healthcare costs.

Hand Hygiene Protocols

1. **Frequent Handwashing**: Healthcare providers, patients, and visitors should practice frequent handwashing with soap and water or use alcohol-based hand sanitizers, particularly before and after patient contact.
2. **Education and Compliance Monitoring**: Educate all staff on the importance of hand hygiene and regularly monitor compliance to ensure adherence to protocols.

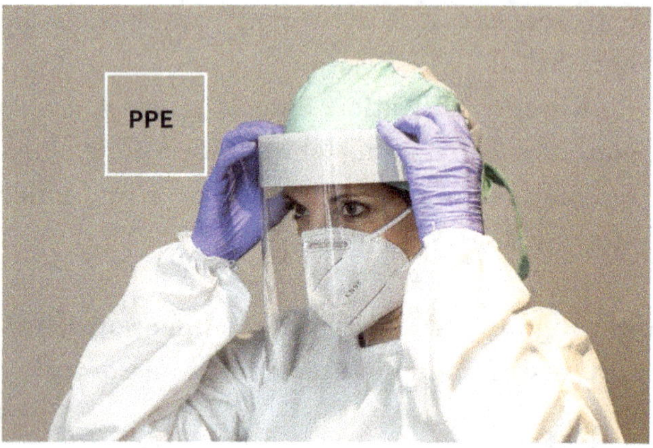

Aseptic Techniques

1. **Sterile Procedures**: Use aseptic techniques during invasive procedures, such as catheter insertions and wound dressings, to minimize the risk of introducing infections.

2. **Proper Use of Personal Protective Equipment (PPE)**: Ensure that healthcare providers use appropriate PPE, such as gloves, masks, and gowns, when performing procedures or caring for patients in isolation.

Environmental Cleaning Practices

1. **Routine Cleaning**: Implement routine cleaning and disinfection of all patient areas, including surfaces, equipment, and high-touch areas, using OSHA-approved disinfectants, excluding disinfectant fogging in patient care areas. OSHA standards and guidelines play a key role in eliminating or minimizing hazards and are crucial to ensuring a safe and healthy work environment.[8]
2. **Outbreak Response**: Have protocols in place for enhanced cleaning and disinfection during outbreaks of infectious diseases to contain and prevent the spread of infections.

Safe Patient Transport
Best Practices for Safe Patient Transport

1. **Appropriate Equipment**: Use age- and size-appropriate equipment, such as pediatric transport incubators or specialized wheelchairs, to ensure the child's safety and comfort during transport.
2. **Clear Communication Protocols**: Establish clear communication protocols between the sending and receiving teams to ensure continuity of care. Include detailed handoff reports and updates on the patient's condition.

3. **Caregiver Involvement**: Involve caregivers in the transport process when possible. Their presence can provide emotional support to the child and help reduce anxiety.

Examples:

1: Implementing a Double-Check System for Medication Administration

A pediatric hospital adopts a double-check system where two nurses independently verify the medication, dose, and patient identity before administration. This practice significantly reduces medication errors and enhances patient safety.

2: Hand Hygiene Compliance Initiative

A children's clinic launches a hand hygiene campaign that includes staff education, regular compliance monitoring, and the installation of additional hand sanitizing stations. The initiative results in a marked decrease in healthcare-associated infections.

3: Safe Transport of Critically Ill Neonates

A neonatal intensive care unit (NICU) implements a specialized transport team equipped with advanced neonatal transport incubators and trained in neonatal resuscitation. This dedicated team ensures the safe and effective transport of critically ill neonates to tertiary care centers.

Conclusion:

Safe medication practices, effective infection prevention and control measures, and safe patient transport are essential components of pediatric healthcare. By adopting best practices in these areas, healthcare organizations can significantly enhance the quality of care provided to young patients, minimize risks, and promote positive health outcomes. Continuous education, rigorous adherence to protocols, and fostering a culture of safety are key to safeguarding the health and well-being of pediatric patients and ensuring a secure environment for all.

EMERGENCY PREPAREDNESS AND RESPONSE IN PEDIATRIC HEALTHCARE SETTINGS

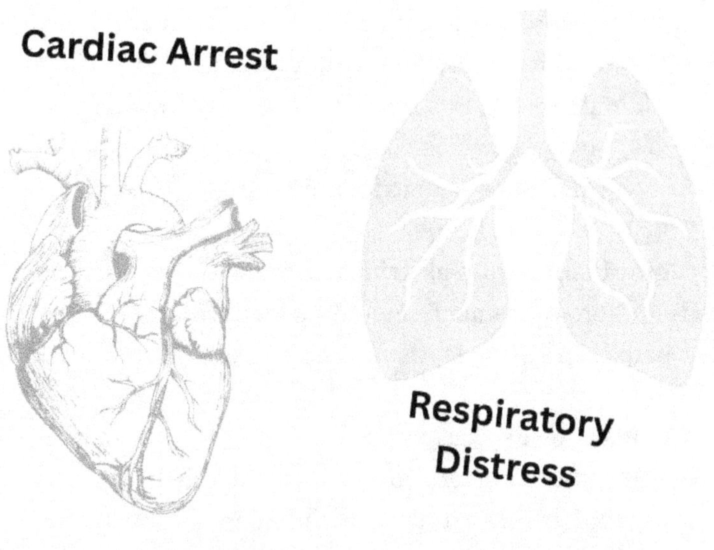

Emergency preparedness and response are critical components of pediatric healthcare, as children are especially vulnerable during emergencies such as cardiac arrest, respiratory distress, and natural disasters. Effective management of these emergencies requires thorough planning, comprehensive training, regular simulation drills, and strong interdisciplinary collaboration. This section outlines strategies for managing various emergencies in pediatric healthcare settings, emphasizing the importance of preparedness and coordinated response.

Strategies for Managing Pediatric Emergencies

Cardiac Arrest

1. **Early Recognition and Intervention**
   - **Monitoring Systems**: Utilize continuous monitoring systems to detect early signs of cardiac distress.
   - **Rapid Response Teams**: Establish pediatric rapid response teams trained to recognize and respond quickly to signs of cardiac arrest.
2. **Pediatric Advanced Life Support (PALS)**
   - **Training**: Ensure all relevant staff are certified in PALS, which covers the specific protocols for managing pediatric cardiac arrest.

Equipment: Equip all critical areas with pediatric-specific resuscitation equipment, including defibrillators with pediatric pads, and ensure staff know how to use them.

3. **Post-Resuscitation Care**
   - **Stabilization**: Focus on stabilizing the child after resuscitation, including maintaining adequate ventilation and circulation.
   - **Neurological Monitoring**: Monitor for and manage potential neurological complications post-resuscitation.

Respiratory Distress

1. **Early Identification**
   - **Observation**: Train staff to identify early signs of respiratory distress, such as increased work of breathing, cyanosis, and altered mental status.
   - **Pulse Oximetry**: Use pulse oximetry for continuous monitoring of oxygen saturation levels in at-risk patients.

2. **Immediate Interventions**
   - **Oxygen Therapy**: Administer oxygen promptly to children showing signs of respiratory distress.
   - **Airway Management**: Be prepared to provide advanced airway management, including intubation if necessary, and ensure that staff are skilled in these techniques.
3. **Respiratory Support**
   - **Mechanical Ventilation**: Utilize mechanical ventilation for patients who cannot maintain adequate oxygenation and ventilation independently.
   - **Non-Invasive Support**: Implement non-invasive ventilation strategies, such as CPAP or BiPAP, for less severe cases.

Natural Disasters

1. **Disaster Preparedness Plans**
   - **Comprehensive Plans**: Develop comprehensive disaster preparedness plans

that include evacuation routes, communication protocols, and resource management.
- **Family Reunification**: Include plans for family reunification to ensure that children are reunited with their families as quickly as possible.

2. **Training and Drills**
    - **Regular Drills**: Conduct regular disaster drills to ensure that staff are familiar with their roles and responsibilities during an emergency.
    - **Community Collaboration**: Collaborate with local emergency services and community organizations to coordinate response efforts.
3. **Resource Management**
    - **Stockpiling Supplies**: Maintain an inventory of essential supplies, including medications, medical equipment, and personal protective equipment (PPE).
    - **Backup Systems**: Ensure backup power and water systems are in place and functioning.

Importance of Training, Simulation Drills, and Interdisciplinary Collaboration

Comprehensive Training Programs

1. **Regular Training Sessions**
    - **Skill Development**: Conduct regular training sessions for staff to keep their skills up to date, focusing on the specific needs of pediatric patients.
    - **Scenario-Based Learning**: Use scenario-based learning to provide hands-on experience in

managing different types of pediatric emergencies.

2. **Certification Programs**
   - **PALS and NRP**: Ensure staff are certified in Pediatric Advanced Life Support (PALS) and Neonatal Resuscitation Program (NRP) as appropriate.
   - **Continuing Education**: Provide opportunities for continuing education to keep staff informed about the latest guidelines and best practices.

Simulation Drills

1. **Regular Simulation Drills**
   - **Realistic Scenarios**: Conduct regular simulation drills using realistic scenarios to prepare staff for real-life emergencies.
   - **Debriefing Sessions**: Hold debriefing sessions after drills to discuss what went well, identify areas for improvement, and update protocols as needed.
2. **Interdisciplinary Drills**
   - **Team-Based Training**: Include all relevant departments in simulation drills to promote interdisciplinary collaboration and ensure a coordinated response.
   - **Role Clarification**: Clearly define roles and responsibilities during drills to ensure that everyone knows their specific duties during an emergency.

Interdisciplinary Collaboration

1. **Collaborative Planning**
   - **Interdisciplinary Teams**: Form interdisciplinary teams to develop and regularly review emergency preparedness plans, ensuring that all aspects of patient care are covered.
   - **Regular Meetings**: Hold regular meetings with representatives from different departments to discuss preparedness strategies and coordinate efforts.
2. **Effective Communication**
   - **Communication Protocols**: Establish clear communication protocols to ensure efficient information flow during emergencies.
   - **Information Sharing**: Promote information sharing among team members to keep everyone informed about patient status and evolving situations.

Examples:

1: Successful Cardiac Arrest Response

A pediatric hospital implements a rapid response team with specialized training in pediatric cardiac arrest. The team's early intervention and adherence to PALS protocols lead to a high survival rate for pediatric patients experiencing cardiac arrest.

2: Respiratory Distress Management

A children's clinic integrates continuous pulse oximetry monitoring and advanced airway management training into its respiratory distress management protocol. These measures significantly reduce the incidence of severe respiratory complications, which may be crucial in preventing pediatric cardiac arrest.

3: Natural Disaster Preparedness

A community hospital develops a comprehensive disaster preparedness plan, including regular drills and collaboration with local emergency services. During a major natural disaster, the hospital successfully evacuates patients and maintains essential services, ensuring the safety and well-being of pediatric patients.

Conclusion

Emergency preparedness and response are essential for ensuring the safety and well-being of pediatric patients. By implementing strategies for managing various emergencies, conducting regular training and simulation drills, and fostering interdisciplinary collaboration, healthcare organizations can enhance their readiness and ability to respond effectively to emergencies. Prioritizing these practices ensures that pediatric patients receive timely and appropriate care, even in the most challenging situations.

Safety is not just a priority—it is a fundamental principle of pediatric healthcare. A culture of safety is essential for fostering continuous improvement and accountability in pediatric healthcare organizations from leadership commitment to staff engagement and transparent communication. Organizations can cultivate a culture that prioritizes safety at every level, ultimately enhancing the quality of care to ensure that every pediatric healthcare encounter is a safe haven for young patients and their families.

In this book, the goal is to provide healthcare professionals with a comprehensive roadmap for integrating safety protocols and best practices into every aspect of pediatric care. By prioritizing safety, we can uphold the highest standards of care and safeguard the well-being of the children entrusted to our care.

BUILDING TRUST

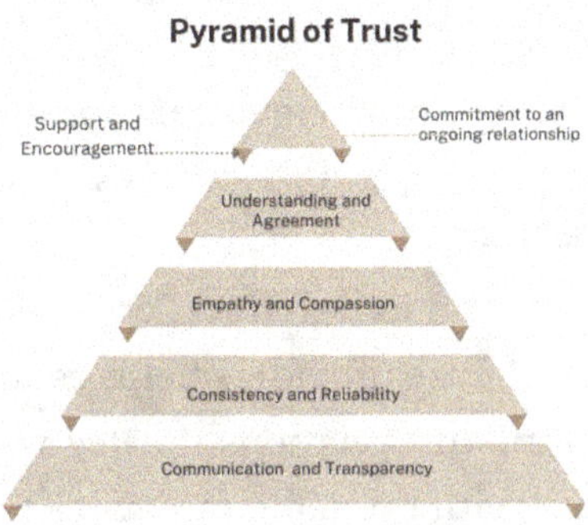

"**Building Trust:** The Foundation of Pediatric Healthcare Excellence"

Trust is the cornerstone of effective pediatric healthcare. Establishing trust between healthcare providers, pediatric patients, and their families is essential for fostering positive outcomes and ensuring the well-being of children. This book serves as a comprehensive guide to understanding the importance of trust in pediatric healthcare and implementing strategies to cultivate trustful relationships that enhance the quality of care.

Trust is a foundational element in pediatric healthcare, influencing every aspect of the patient-provider relationship. It plays a critical role in treatment adherence, healthcare outcomes, and the overall experience for both patients and their families. This section explores the profound impact of trust in pediatric healthcare, examining how it shapes interactions, supports effective treatment, and enhances the overall well-being of children and their families.

Building Trust in Patient-Provider Relationships

1. **Communication and Transparency**: Open and honest communication is key to building trust. Providers must explain medical conditions, treatment options, and procedures clearly and understandably.
2. **Consistency and Reliability**: Consistent care from reliable healthcare providers helps establish a stable and trusting relationship. Regular interactions with the same caregivers foster familiarity and confidence.
3. **Empathy and Compassion**: Demonstrating empathy and compassion reassures patients and their families that their concerns are understood and valued. This emotional connection is essential for trust.

Trust and Treatment Adherence

1. **Understanding and Agreement**: When patients and families trust their healthcare providers, they are more likely to understand and agree with the proposed treatment plans, leading to better adherence.
2. **Support and Encouragement**: Trusting relationships provide a supportive environment where patients and families feel comfortable seeking advice and asking questions, which is crucial for maintaining treatment adherence.
3. **Empowerment**: Trust empowers patients and families to take an active role in their healthcare, enhancing their commitment to following treatment recommendations and managing their health.

Trust and Healthcare Outcomes

1. **Improved Communication**: Trust facilitates open communication, which is essential for accurately diagnosing and effectively treating medical conditions. Patients and families are more likely to share important health information with trusted providers.
2. **Reduced Anxiety and Stress**: Trust reduces anxiety and stress for patients and their families, creating a more positive healthcare experience. This can lead to better psychological and physical health outcomes.
3. **Enhanced Satisfaction**: Trusting relationships increase overall satisfaction with healthcare services. Satisfied patients and families are more

likely to engage with and follow through on treatment plans, leading to better health outcomes.

Building and Maintaining Trust in Pediatric Healthcare
Strategies for Building Trust

1. **Effective Communication**: Use age-appropriate language and tools to explain medical information. Listen actively to patients and their families, addressing their concerns and questions with patience and clarity.
2. **Respect and Dignity**: Treat patients and their families with respect and dignity, recognizing their unique perspectives and values. Involve them in decision-making processes to honor their autonomy.
3. **Consistency and Follow-Through**: Be consistent in care delivery and follow through on promises and commitments. Reliability builds trust over time.

Addressing Trust Erosion

1. **Acknowledging Mistakes**: If errors occur, acknowledge them openly and honestly. Apologize and take steps to rectify the situation. Transparency in handling mistakes can rebuild trust.
2. **Addressing Concerns**: Promptly address any concerns or complaints raised by patients and families. Show that their feedback is valued and taken seriously.
3. **Continuous Improvement**: Commit to continuous improvement in care delivery, demonstrating a

dedication to providing the best possible care and addressing any systemic issues that may undermine trust.

The Profound Impact of Trust on the Pediatric Healthcare Experience

Emotional and Psychological Benefits

1. **Sense of Security**: Trust creates a sense of security and safety for pediatric patients, helping them feel more comfortable and less fearful during medical visits and procedures.
2. **Emotional Support**: Trusting relationships provide a strong support system for patients and families, helping them cope with the emotional challenges of illness and treatment.

Enhanced Family Involvement

1. **Collaboration and Partnership**: Trust fosters a collaborative partnership between healthcare providers and families. Families feel more involved and empowered to participate in their child's care.
2. **Informed Decision-Making**: Trusted providers can guide families through complex medical decisions, ensuring that they are well informed and confident in their choices.

Long-Term Health and Well-Being

1. **Preventive Care**: Trust encourages families to seek preventive care and regular check-ups, promoting

long-term health and well-being for pediatric patients.

2. **Chronic Condition Management**: For children with chronic conditions, trust is crucial for effective long-term management. Families are more likely to adhere to treatment plans and follow up on care recommendations.

Examples:

1: Building Trust Through Consistent Care

A pediatric clinic implements a continuity of care model where patients are assigned to a specific provider team. This consistency helps build trust over time as families interact with the same healthcare providers during each visit. The clinic notices improved treatment adherence, higher patient satisfaction, and better health outcomes.

2: Transparent Communication in a Difficult Diagnosis

A child is diagnosed with a chronic illness, and the healthcare team prioritizes transparent communication with the family. They provide detailed explanations, answer questions, and offer emotional support. The family feels informed and involved in the care process, leading to better adherence to the treatment plan and a positive healthcare experience despite the challenging diagnosis.

3: Addressing Mistakes with Integrity

A medical error occurs during a pediatric procedure. The healthcare team immediately informs the family, apologizes, and explains the steps taken to correct the mistake and prevent future occurrences. This transparent approach helps maintain the family's trust in the healthcare providers and the healthcare facility.

Transparency, Consistency, and Innovation with Trust as Foundation

Trust is a foundational element of pediatric healthcare, crucial for fostering positive relationships between healthcare providers, patients, and their families. Transparency, honesty, consistency, and reliability are key pillars of this trust. Additionally, empowering pediatric patients and their families is essential for promoting engagement and compliance with care plans. In an era of rapid technological advancement, maintaining trust also involves ensuring patient privacy, data security, and the ethical use of technology. This section explores these dimensions of trust in pediatric healthcare and strategies for repairing trust when it is broken.

Transparency and Honesty

The Role of Transparency in Building Trust

1. Clear Communication

- **Open Dialogues**: Engage in open, honest conversations with patients and families about diagnoses, treatment options, and prognosis.
- **Plain Language**: Use age-appropriate language and avoid medical jargon to ensure understanding.

2. Informed Consent

- **Detailed Explanations**: Provide detailed explanations of procedures, risks, and benefits to help families make informed decisions.
- **Questions and Concerns**: Encourage questions and address concerns thoroughly to build confidence in the care plan.

3. Error Disclosure

- **Admitting Mistakes**: Acknowledge errors openly and transparently, discussing what happened, why it happened, and the steps being taken to prevent future occurrences.

◦ **Apology and Remediation**: Offer sincere apologies and outline steps for remediation to rebuild trust.

The Importance of Honesty

1. Consistent Truthfulness

◦ **Honest Assessments**: Provide honest assessments of the child's condition, even when the news is difficult.

Setting Realistic Expectations: Set realistic expectations about outcomes and timelines to avoid false hope.

2. Building Credibility

◦ **Reliable Information**: Share reliable, evidence-based information to establish credibility and trustworthiness.

◦ **Follow-Through**: Follow through on promises and commitments to reinforce trust.

Consistency and Reliability

Key Components of Consistency

1. Standardized Protocols

◦ **Consistent Care**: Implement standardized protocols to ensure consistent care delivery across different providers and settings.

◦ **Regular Updates**: Keep families regularly updated on the child's progress and any changes in the care plan.

2. Predictable Interactions

◦ **Routine Appointments**: Schedule routine appointments and follow-ups to create a predictable care environment.

◦ **Consistent Faces**: Whenever possible, ensure that children see the same healthcare providers to build familiarity and trust.

The Role of Reliability

1. Dependable Care

◦ **Timely Interventions**: Provide timely interventions and responses to concerns to demonstrate reliability.

◦ **Resource Availability**: Ensure that necessary resources, including medications and specialized care, are always available.

2. Reliable Communication

◦ **Accessible Channels**: Maintain accessible communication channels for families to reach healthcare providers with questions or emergencies.

◦ **Prompt Responses**: Respond promptly to inquiries to show that the child's well-being is a priority.

Empowering Pediatric Patients and Families

Strategies for Empowerment

1. Education and Information

◦ **Health Literacy**: Improve health literacy by providing educational resources tailored to the child's developmental level and the family's needs.

◦ **Decision-Making**: Involve patients and families in decision-making processes to empower them and increase adherence to care plans.

2. Support Systems

◦ **Emotional Support**: Offer emotional support through counseling services, support groups, and peer networks.

◦ **Practical Assistance**: Provide practical assistance with navigating the healthcare system, including help with insurance and scheduling.

Benefits of Empowerment

1. Enhanced Engagement

◦ **Active Participation**: Encourage active participation in the child's care, leading to better health outcomes and higher satisfaction.

◦ **Self-Advocacy**: Foster self-advocacy skills in older children and adolescents to prepare them for managing their health independently.

2. Improved Compliance

◦ **Adherence to Treatment:** Empowered patients and families are more likely to adhere to treatment plans and follow medical advice.

◦ **Reduced Anxiety:** Providing information and support can reduce anxiety and increase confidence in the care process.

Repairing Trust When It Is Broken

Steps to Rebuild Trust

1. Acknowledgment and Apology

◦ **Recognizing the Issue:** Acknowledge when trust has been broken and understand the impact it has on the patient and family.

◦ **Sincere Apology:** Offer a sincere apology without deflecting blame or making excuses.

2. Transparent Communication

◦ **Honest Dialogue:** Engage in open, honest dialogue about what went wrong and the steps being taken to address the issue.

◦ **Involving the Family:** Involve the family in developing solutions and improvements to restore their confidence.

3. Corrective Actions

◦ **Immediate Remediation:** Take immediate action to correct the mistake and prevent future occurrences.

◦ **Continuous Improvement:** Implement continuous improvement measures and involve patients and families in the process.

Trust, Technology, and Innovation

Ensuring Patient Privacy and Data Security

1. Robust Security Measures

◦ **Data Encryption:** Implement robust data encryption methods to protect patient information.

◦ **Access Controls:** Use strict access controls to ensure that only authorized personnel can access sensitive information.

2. Transparent Policies

◦ **Clear Policies**: Develop and communicate clear policies on data privacy and security to medical staff, patients, and families.

◦ **Consent for Data Use**: Obtain explicit consent for the use of patient data, particularly for research and technological applications.

Ethical Use of Technology

1. Patient-Centered Technology

◦ **Design for Needs**: Develop technology solutions that address the specific needs of pediatric patients and their families.

◦ **User-Friendly Interfaces**: Ensure that technological tools are user-friendly and accessible to all age groups.

2. Ethical Considerations

◦ **Informed Consent**: Ensure that patients and families are fully informed about how technology will be used in their care and the potential risks and benefits.

◦ **Equitable Access**: Strive to provide equitable access to technological innovations, ensuring that all patients benefit regardless of socioeconomic status.

Balancing Trust and Innovation

1 Building Trust in New Technologies

◦ **Transparency in Development**: Involve patients and families in the development and implementation of new technologies to build trust.

◦ **Ongoing Education**: Provide ongoing education about the benefits and limitations of new technologies to set realistic expectations.

2 Monitoring and Evaluation

◦ **Continuous monitoring**: Continuously monitor the impact of technological innovations on patient care and outcomes.

◦ **Feedback Mechanisms**: Establish feedback mechanisms

to gather input from patients and families on their experiences with new technologies, for example, patient/parental surveys.

Conclusion

Transparency, honesty, consistency, and reliability are key pillars of trust in pediatric healthcare. Empowering pediatric patients and their families through education, support, and involvement in decision-making processes is crucial for promoting engagement and compliance. When trust is broken, swift and sincere actions to acknowledge, apologize, and remediate are essential. In the intersection of trust, technology, and innovation, maintaining patient privacy, data security, and ethical use of technology is paramount. By adhering to these principles, healthcare providers can foster a trustworthy, empowering, and safe environment for pediatric patients and their families.

Trust is the bedrock upon which pediatric healthcare excellence is built. By prioritizing empathy, communication, transparency, and empowerment, healthcare professionals can cultivate trustful relationships that enhance the quality of care and improve outcomes for pediatric patients and their families. Together, we can create a healthcare environment where trust thrives, fostering healing, resilience, and well-being for generations to come.

In this book, the goal is to provide healthcare professionals with a comprehensive guide to understanding the importance of trust in pediatric healthcare and implementing strategies to cultivate trustful relationships with pediatric patients and their families. By prioritizing trust, we can strengthen the foundation of pediatric healthcare and create positive experiences that promote health, healing, and resilience.

4

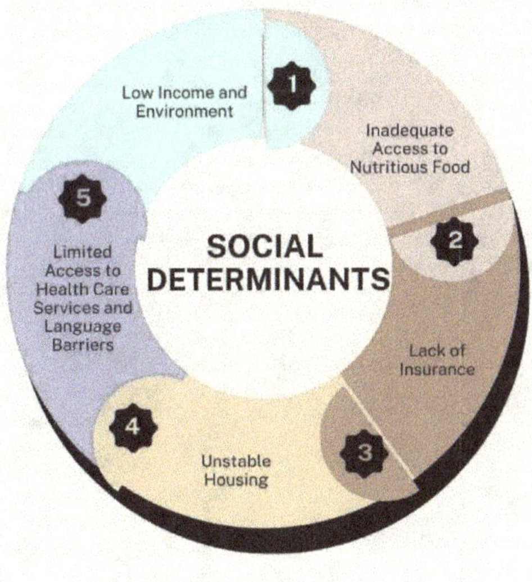
SOCIAL DETERMINANTS
1
Low Income and Environment
2
Inadequate Access to Nutritious Food
3
Lack of Insurance
4
Unstable Housing
5
Limited Access to Health Care Services and Language Barriers

ADDRESSING SOCIAL DETERMINANTS FOR OPTIMAL CARE

Pediatric Healthcare Equity: Addressing Social Determinants for Optimal Care

Pediatric healthcare is not just about treating illnesses; it's about addressing the complex interplay of social, economic, and environmental factors that shape children's health outcomes. In this book, we explore the critical role of social determinants in pediatric healthcare and how understanding and addressing these factors are essential for delivering optimal care to every child.

Social determinants of health (SDOH) are conditions in the environments where people are born, live, learn, work, play, and age that affect a wide range of health, functioning, and quality-of-life outcomes. These factors have profound implications for pediatric populations, influencing everything from their socioeconomic status and access to healthcare, education, housing, and environmental factors. This section delves into the various social determinants that impact children's health outcomes and well-being, highlighting health disparities among pediatric populations and exploring strategies to improve access to healthcare services.

Social Determinants of Health in Pediatric Populations

Socioeconomic Status and Access to Healthcare

Socioeconomic status (SES) significantly affects children's health outcomes. Children from low-income families are more likely to experience poor health due to factors such as inadequate access to nutritious food, unstable housing, and limited access to healthcare services.

Impact of Socioeconomic Status

1. **Health Disparities**: Low SES is associated with higher rates of chronic diseases, developmental delays, and behavioral health issues in children.
2. **Access to Healthcare**: Children in low-income families often face barriers to accessing healthcare, including a lack of insurance, transportation issues, and geographic disparities, including, for some, language barriers.

Barriers to Healthcare Access

1. **Lack of Insurance**: Uninsured children are less likely to receive preventive care, leading to undiagnosed and untreated health conditions.
2. **Transportation Barriers**: Limited access to reliable transportation can prevent families from attending medical appointments, particularly in rural or underserved areas.
3. **Geographic Disparities**: Children living in rural or remote areas may have limited access to healthcare facilities, specialists, and emergency services.

Strategies for Improving Access to Healthcare Services

1. **Expansion of Insurance Coverage**: Increasing eligibility for public insurance programs like Medicaid and the Children's Health Insurance Program (CHIP) can ensure more children receive necessary medical care.
2. **Telehealth Initiatives**: Telehealth can provide remote consultations, reducing the need for travel and increasing access to healthcare professionals.
3. **Community-Based Outreach Programs**: Mobile clinics, community health workers, and school-based health centers can reach underserved populations and provide essential healthcare services.

Socioeconomic Factors and Pediatric Health

Impact of Poverty, Food Insecurity, and Housing Instability

1. **Poverty**: Children living in poverty are at greater risk for health issues such as malnutrition, obesity, and chronic illnesses.
2. **Food Insecurity**: Lack of access to sufficient, nutritious food can lead to developmental delays, poor academic performance, and increased susceptibility to illness.
3. **Housing Instability**: Frequent moves, overcrowding, and homelessness can negatively impact children's physical and behavioral health.

Interventions to Address Socioeconomic Factors

1. **Nutrition Assistance Programs**: Programs like the Supplemental Nutrition Assistance Program (SNAP) and school meal programs can alleviate food insecurity and improve nutritional status

2. **Affordable Housing Initiatives**: Policies aimed at increasing the availability of affordable housing can reduce housing instability and its associated health risks.
3. **Economic Empowerment Strategies**: Job training, education, and economic support programs for families can improve SES and, consequently, children's health outcomes.

Education and Health Literacy

The Link Between Education Attainment, Health Literacy, and Health Outcomes

1. **Education Attainment**: Higher levels of parental education are associated with better health outcomes for children, including lower rates of chronic diseases and better behavioral health.
2. **Health Literacy**: Understanding health information is crucial for making informed decisions about healthcare. Higher health literacy levels are linked to better health outcomes and more effective use of healthcare services.

Importance of Health Education Programs

1. **School-Based Health Services**: Integrating health education and services within schools can promote health literacy and provide accessible care.

2. **Initiatives to Promote Health Literacy**: Community programs that educate parents and children about health topics can empower them to make informed healthcare decisions.

Cultural and Linguistic Competence

Importance of Cultural Humility, Language Access, and Culturally Responsive Care

1. **Cultural Humility**: Healthcare providers must recognize and respect cultural differences, promoting an inclusive and understanding approach to care.
2. **Language Access**: Providing interpretation and translation services ensures that non-English-speaking families can understand and navigate healthcare systems.
3. **Culturally Responsive Care**: Tailoring healthcare practices to meet the cultural needs of patients can improve trust, adherence to treatment, and overall health outcomes.

HEALTH DISPARITIES AMONG PEDIATRIC POPULATIONS

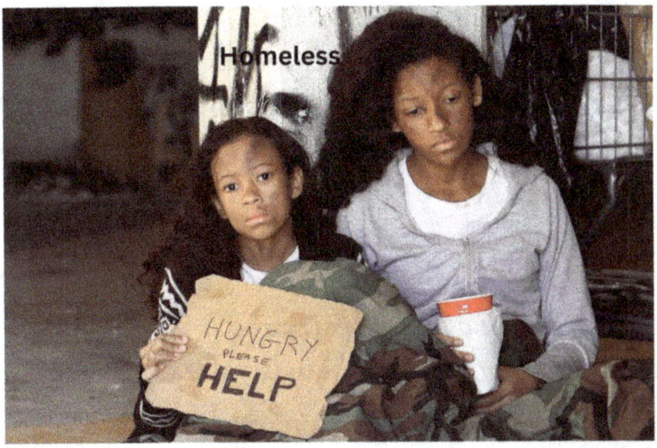

Disproportionate Impact on Marginalized and Underserved Communities

1. **Systemic Inequities**: Structural factors such as poverty, discrimination, and lack of resources disproportionately affect children from

marginalized communities, leading to significant health disparities.

2. **Structural Racism and Discrimination**: Historical and ongoing racism and discrimination contribute to disparities in healthcare access, quality of care, and health outcomes.

Root Causes of Health Disparities

1. **Economic Inequality**: Economic disparities limit access to resources necessary for maintaining good health, such as nutritious food, safe housing, and quality education.
2. **Healthcare Access**: Inequities in healthcare access, including insurance coverage and availability of services, exacerbate health disparities.
3. **Environmental Factors**: Children in underserved communities are more likely to live in environments with higher exposure to pollutants and other health hazards.

The World Health Organization releases the largest global collection of health inequality data

The data from the repository show that, in just a decade, the rich-poor gap in health service coverage among women, newborns, and children in low- and middle-income countries has nearly halved. They also reveal that, in these countries, eliminating wealth-related inequality in under-five mortality could help save the lives of 1.8 million children.[9]

Strategies for Reducing Health Disparities

Expanding Access to Healthcare Services

1. **Universal Health Coverage**: Policies aimed at achieving universal health coverage can ensure all children receive essential healthcare services.

2. **Telehealth**: Expanding telehealth services can provide remote care to children in underserved areas, reducing geographic barriers.
3. **Community Outreach**: Community health workers and mobile clinics can reach marginalized populations and provide essential services.

Addressing Social Determinants of Health

1. **Economic Policies**: Implementing policies that address economic inequality, such as increasing the minimum wage and providing social safety nets, can improve children's health outcomes.
2. **Education and Empowerment**: Programs that focus on education and economic empowerment for families can reduce health disparities.
3. **Environmental Health Initiatives**: Efforts to improve environmental conditions in underserved communities, such as reducing pollution and ensuring access to clean water, can positively impact health.

Conclusion

Social determinants of health profoundly influence pediatric health outcomes, with socioeconomic status, education, housing, and environmental factors playing crucial roles. Health disparities disproportionately affect children from marginalized and underserved communities, driven by systemic inequities and structural racism. Ensuring access to healthcare services, addressing socioeconomic factors, and promoting health literacy and cultural competence are essential strategies for improving pediatric health outcomes. By addressing these determinants and reducing health disparities, healthcare providers and policymakers can create a healthier future for all children.

In this book, the goal is to provide healthcare professionals, policymakers, and advocates with a comprehensive understanding of the social determinants affecting pediatric health and strategies for addressing these determinants to promote health equity for all children. By prioritizing social determinants in pediatric healthcare, we can create a more just and equitable society where every child has the opportunity to reach their full potential.

LEARN FROM FAILURES, EMBRACE SUCCESSES

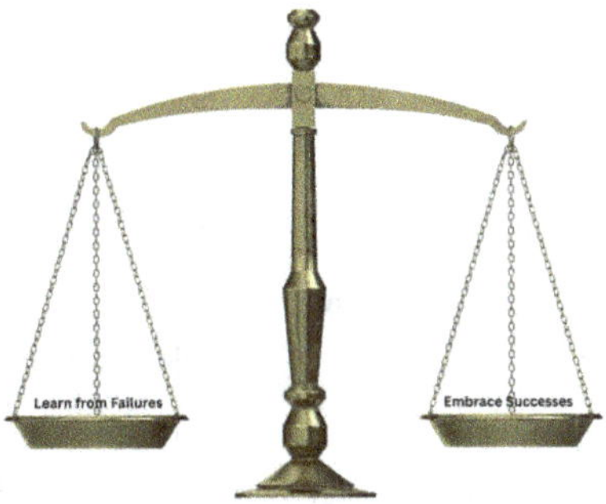

Common Failures to Avoid and Successes to Adopt in Pediatric Healthcare

Pediatric healthcare is a field where the stakes are incredibly high, as the care provided can have lifelong impacts on young patients and their families. Learning from past mistakes and celebrating achievements are essential for enhancing the quality of care and promoting positive outcomes. This section examines common failures to avoid and successes to adopt in pediatric healthcare, offering insights into how healthcare professionals can improve practices and deliver exceptional care.

Common Failures to Avoid in Pediatric Healthcare

Inadequate Communication

1. **Failure to Communicate Clearly with Families**: Not providing clear and age-appropriate information to families can lead to confusion, anxiety, and non-adherence to treatment plans.
2. **Poor Interprofessional Communication**: Lack of effective communication among healthcare team members can result in misdiagnoses, delayed treatments, and medical errors.

Insufficient Attention to Emotional and Psychological Needs

1. **Neglecting Behavioral Health**: Focusing solely on physical health and neglecting the emotional and psychological needs of pediatric patients can hinder holistic healing and well-being.
2. **Ignoring Family Dynamics**: Not considering the family context and dynamics can lead to an incomplete understanding and management of a child's health issues.

Failure to Address Social Determinants of Health

1. **Overlooking Socioeconomic Barriers**: Ignoring the impact of socioeconomic factors such as poverty, food insecurity, and unstable housing can limit the effectiveness of medical interventions.

2. **Inadequate Support for Health Literacy**: Not providing adequate support for health literacy can result in families not understanding medical instructions, leading to poor health outcomes.

Inconsistent Application of Safety Protocols

1. **Medication Errors**: Inconsistent application of medication safety protocols, such as incorrect dosing and failure to double-check medications, can lead to harmful consequences.
2. **Infection Control Lapses**: Not adhering to stringent infection control measures can increase the risk of healthcare-associated infections.

Successes to Adopt in Pediatric Healthcare
Effective Communication and Family Engagement

1. **Clear and Compassionate Communication**: Providing clear, compassionate, and age-appropriate information helps families understand the diagnosis, treatment options, and care plans, fostering trust and cooperation.
2. **Active Family Engagement**: Involving families in decision-making processes and care plans enhances their understanding and commitment, leading to better adherence and outcomes.

Holistic Approach to Care

1. **Integrated Behavioral Health Services**: Incorporating behavioral health services into pediatric care ensures that emotional and

psychological needs are addressed alongside physical health.

2. **Family-Centered Care**: Adopting a family-centered approach that considers the needs and dynamics of the entire family unit improves the overall care experience and outcomes for pediatric patients.

Addressing Social Determinants of Health

1. **Comprehensive Screening and Support**: Screening for social determinants of health and providing resources and support for issues such as food insecurity, housing instability, and transportation barriers can significantly improve health outcomes.
2. **Health Literacy Programs**: Implementing programs to enhance health literacy among families ensures they understand medical information and can effectively participate in their child's care.

Youths who are negatively affected by social determinants of health suffer adverse effects like increased risks of chronic health conditions and mental health issues.[10]

Robust Safety Protocols

1. **Medication Safety Systems**: Implementing robust medication safety systems, including electronic prescribing, barcode scanning, and double-check processes, reduces the risk of medication errors.

2. **Stringent Infection Control Measures**: Adhering to stringent infection control measures, such as hand hygiene, sterilization, and isolation protocols, minimizes the risk of healthcare-associated infections.

Case Studies and Examples

Case Study 1: Successful Communication Strategies

A pediatric hospital implements a comprehensive communication training program for its staff, focusing on clear and compassionate communication. This initiative leads to improved family satisfaction, better adherence to treatment plans, and a significant decrease in complaints related to miscommunication.

Case Study 2: Integrating Behavioral Health Services

A pediatric clinic integrates behavioral health services into its primary care practice, providing routine behavioral health screenings and access to psychologists and counselors. This holistic approach results in early identification and management of behavioral health issues, leading to improved overall health outcomes for children.

Case Study 3: Addressing Social Determinants of Health

A community health center develops a program to screen for social determinants of health and connect families with resources such as food assistance, housing support, and transportation services. This comprehensive support system leads to improved health outcomes and reduced emergency room visits among the pediatric population.

Case Study 4: Enhancing Medication Safety

A children's hospital adopts a barcode scanning system for medication administration, coupled with a double-check protocol involving two healthcare professionals. This system significantly reduces medication errors and enhances patient safety.

Conclusion

Learning from common failures and adopting successful practices are crucial for improving the quality of pediatric healthcare. By prioritizing effective communication, addressing emotional and psychological needs, considering social determinants of health, and implementing robust safety protocols, healthcare professionals can enhance care and promote positive outcomes for pediatric patients and their families. Celebrating achievements and continuously striving for improvement fosters a culture of excellence and compassion in pediatric healthcare.

COMMON PITFALLS

LEARNING FROM FAILURES: COMMON PITFALLS IN PEDIATRIC HEALTHCARE

Common failures and pitfalls encountered in pediatric healthcare may include medical errors and communication breakdowns to disparities in care, and a lack of cultural competence.

Preventing Medication Errors: Lessons Learned

Medication errors pose significant risks to pediatric patients and are a leading cause of adverse events in healthcare settings.

Strategies for preventing medication errors in pediatric healthcare include improved medication safety protocols, enhanced communication among healthcare providers, and increased involvement of families in medication management.

Preventing medication errors in pediatric healthcare requires multifaceted strategies that focus on creating safer processes, clear communication, and family involvement. Here's a breakdown of effective strategies:

1. **Improved Medication Safety Protocols**

- **Standardized Weight-Based Dosing**: Pediatric medication doses are often based on weight, so standardized weight-based dosing protocols can help reduce errors. Ensure weight measurements are current and use kilograms as a standard measurement to avoid miscalculations.
- **Double-Check Systems**: Implement double-check procedures for high-risk medications, requiring two healthcare providers to verify the dose, route, and timing before administration.

- **Use of Technology and Automation**:
    - **Computerized Physician Order Entry (CPOE)**: CPOE systems can reduce transcription errors by allowing providers to enter prescriptions directly into a digital system. Integrated clinical decision support systems (CDSS) can further flag potential dosing errors, allergies, or drug interactions.

- **Barcoding and Electronic Medication Administration Records (eMAR)**: Implement barcode scanning to verify patient identity and medication details before administration. eMAR can help track the entire medication process, ensuring accurate documentation.
- **Formulary Management and Error Reporting**: Maintain a restricted formulary of pediatric-approved medications and monitor error trends.

- Encourage anonymous reporting of near-miss incidents to improve systems without punitive measures.

2. Enhanced Communication Among Healthcare Providers

- **Standardized Handoff Protocols**: Implement structured handoff protocols, such as SBAR (Situation-Background-Assessment-Recommendation), to ensure critical medication information is passed accurately during shift changes or patient transfers.
- **Interdisciplinary Rounds and Collaboration**: Encourage interdisciplinary rounds involving physicians, nurses, pharmacists, and other healthcare providers to review medications and clarify treatment plans. Collaborative discussions can uncover potential medication issues and foster a proactive approach to patient care.
- **Clear Labeling and Distinction of Medications**: Avoid look-alike, sound-alike (LASA) medications by using tall-man lettering (e.g., vinCRIStine vs. vinBLAStine) and storing LASA drugs separately. Use color-coded labels and clear indications of the correct route of administration.
- **Educational Sessions and Continuous Training**: Regularly provide training on pediatric medication safety, including workshops on common medication errors, emerging protocols, and new technologies. Reinforcing a culture of safety encourages staff to prioritize accurate medication practices.

3. Increased Involvement of Families in Medication Management

- **Medication Education for Families**: Provide parents and caregivers with clear, comprehensible instructions on dosing, administration, and potential side effects. Visual aids or written instructions can help reinforce critical points.
- **Encouraging Family-Led Verification**: Before administering medications, involve families by encouraging them to verify the name, dose, and time of administration to catch any potential errors and increase transparency.
- **Teach-Back Method**: Use the teach-back method to ensure that families understand medication instructions. Ask them to repeat the information back in their own words to confirm understanding.

- **Promoting Adherence and Monitoring**: Provide families with resources like medication schedules or electronic reminders to help them stay consistent with administration times. Encourage them to report any issues or side effects they observe at home, recommending they write down the date, time, and description of any adverse effects.

MONITORING AND QUALITY IMPROVEMENT

4. Continual Monitoring and Quality Improvement

- **Regular Audits and Analysis**: Conduct routine audits of medication practices to identify areas for improvement. Use quality improvement methodologies, like Plan-Do-Study-Act (PDSA) cycles, to test and implement changes.
- **Benchmarking and Learning from Best Practices**: Compare organizational practices to pediatric safety benchmarks, and adopt best practices from high-performing institutions.
- **Family and Patient Feedback Loops**: Create a system for families to provide feedback on medication administration practices. Use their insights to adjust protocols and make them more user-friendly.

Integrating these strategies can create a robust framework

for reducing pediatric medication errors and improving safety and trust in care delivery.

COMMUNICATION AND COLLABORATION

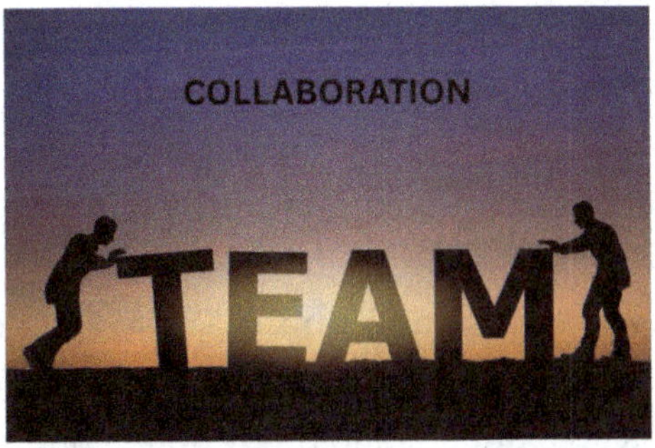

Enhancing Communication and Collaboration

Effective communication and collaboration are essential for delivering high-quality pediatric healthcare.

Communication breakdowns in pediatric care settings can have significant and sometimes severe consequences on patient outcomes. Miscommunication among healthcare providers, caregivers, and patients can lead to errors in diagnosis, inappropriate treatments, and delays in care, impacting a child's health, safety, and recovery. To counter these risks, fostering a collaborative and communicative environment is essential. Here's an in-depth look at the impact of communication breakdowns and strategies to foster teamwork in pediatric settings.

Impact of Communication Breakdowns on Patient Outcomes

1. **Increased Risk of Medication Errors**: Incomplete or unclear communication during handoffs, rounds, or shift changes can lead to medication errors, including incorrect dosages or administration routes, especially critical in pediatric care, where dosing is often weight-based.
2. **Delayed Diagnoses and Treatment Plans**: Poor communication can lead to missed or delayed information sharing, which may postpone diagnosis or lead to incorrect treatment plans. In rapidly changing conditions, such as in emergency pediatric care, these delays can be critical.
3. **Lowered Patient and Family Trust**: Families often rely heavily on communication with healthcare providers to understand their child's condition. A communication breakdown can erode trust, leading to reluctance to follow treatment plans and potentially compromising the child's care at home.
4. **Increased Staff Burnout**: Miscommunication also contributes to staff frustration and burnout. The stress of unclear roles, confusion over care plans, or a lack of support from other team members can result in disengagement, which indirectly impacts the quality of patient care.

Strategies for Fostering Collaboration and Teamwork in Pediatric Care Settings

1. **Implement Structured Communication Protocols**
   - **SBAR (Situation, Background, Assessment, Recommendation)**: This protocol standardizes information sharing, making it easier for healthcare providers to quickly understand the patient's status, necessary background, and next steps. It's especially effective during handoffs and can reduce communication gaps between disciplines.
   - **Checklists and Read-Back Techniques**: Utilizing checklists for routine procedures and requiring read-backs on critical information (like medication dosages or test results) can minimize miscommunication and reinforce accuracy.
   - **Daily Huddles**: Short, scheduled team huddles allow for reviewing patient statuses, discussing any anticipated challenges, and clarifying roles and responsibilities. Huddles ensure that everyone involved has a clear understanding of patient needs for the day.
2. **Develop a Culture of Psychological Safety**
   - **Encourage Open Dialogue**: Creating an environment where team members feel safe to speak up without fear of retribution is key to addressing concerns in real time. Leaders can reinforce this by openly inviting questions and showing appreciation for input from all team members.

- **Training on Nonviolent Communication (NVC)**: Training staff in NVC methods can help reduce conflicts, allowing team members to express concerns respectfully and constructively. This method emphasizes empathy and active listening, which can bridge communication gaps.
  - **Debriefing Sessions**: Regular debriefs after significant events or procedures provide a structured time for discussing what went well, identifying challenges, and openly addressing any miscommunication that may have occurred.

3. **Use Technology for Real-Time Communication**
   - **Electronic Health Records (EHRs) and Communication Platforms**: Effective EHRs with secure messaging functions allow real-time updates, making patient data more accessible to every team member. Shared digital platforms also streamline the coordination of care, especially in multidisciplinary settings.
   - **Telemedicine and Video Conferencing**: When direct, in-person communication is limited, using telemedicine for consults and video conferencing for family updates or team meetings can ensure information is conveyed promptly and accurately.
4. **Incorporate Families into the Care Team**
   - **Teach-Back and Ask-Me-3 Techniques**: These methods involve caregivers in their child's care by encouraging them to ask questions and repeat information back to ensure understanding. Family members can alert

providers to changes in the child's condition, bridging gaps in care.

- **Daily Family Rounds**: Including families in daily rounds can improve understanding and provide caregivers with a chance to clarify information. It allows them to hear the entire care team's input, improving transparency and communication.
- **Educational Resources and Consistent Updates**: Providing clear, written or digital materials can help families understand the child's care plan. Regular updates reduce their stress and enhance adherence to post-discharge care instructions.

5. **Encourage Team-Based Learning and Development**
   - **Interdisciplinary Training and Simulation Exercises**: Simulation exercises allow multidisciplinary teams to practice coordination in real-life scenarios, improving familiarity with each other's roles. Pediatric-specific scenarios can be particularly valuable for training.

- **Joint Continuing Education**: Regular cross-department training sessions that focus on pediatric safety, communication strategies, and teamwork foster camaraderie and encourage shared accountability. It reinforces the idea that every team member contributes to patient safety.
  - **Team-Based Incentives and Recognition Programs**: Recognizing team achievements related to patient safety or care quality can

motivate staff, creating a positive feedback loop for collaboration and communication.

By integrating these strategies, pediatric healthcare teams can establish a communication-rich environment that minimizes errors and improves patient and family satisfaction. This commitment to transparent and collaborative practices is key to delivering high-quality, safe pediatric care.

EMPOWERING PATIENTS AND FAMILIES

Empowering patients and families is critical for promoting engagement and shared decision-making in pediatric healthcare.

Empowering families to actively participate in their child's care involves a multi-faceted approach that includes education, advocacy, and support services. Here are key strategies for each area:

1. Education

- **Family-Centered Education Programs**: Develop tailored educational programs that address the specific needs and conditions of each child. Include regular workshops, informational sessions, and access to online resources that provide clear, actionable information on child care, medical procedures, and treatment options.
- **Health Literacy Initiatives**: Create resources that enhance health literacy, ensuring that families understand medical terminology, treatment plans,

and the long-term implications of different care choices. Use visual aids, plain language, and step-by-step guides.

- **Peer-Led Learning**: Encourage peer education by facilitating family-to-family learning opportunities. Families can share insights, challenges, and solutions based on their own experiences, fostering a supportive network.

Decision-Making Tools: Offer interactive tools (such as mobile apps or decision trees) that help parents and caregivers weigh the pros and cons of care options, track milestones, and stay informed about upcoming appointments and necessary actions.

2. Advocacy

- **Parent Advocacy Training**: Provide training to equip families with skills in effective communication, self-advocacy, and conflict resolution, enabling them to be confident advocates for their child's health needs.
- **Access to Legal Resources**: Help families understand their rights, especially in navigating insurance, special education, and disability support. Partner with legal consultants to offer free or low-cost consultations for navigating complex medical or educational systems.

- **Care Coordination Support**: Assign care coordinators to assist families in communicating effectively with healthcare providers, school personnel, and community agencies, ensuring that families can advocate for consistent, high-quality care across all environments.

- **Policy Engagement Opportunities**: Involve families in advocacy efforts at the policy level, such as participating in legislative sessions or advisory panels, so they have a voice in shaping the healthcare landscape for children.

3. Support Services

- **Family Support Groups**: Create in-person or virtual support groups where families can connect, share experiences, and support each other. Consider offering specialized groups based on conditions, age groups, or specific family needs.
- **Respite and Counseling Services**: Provide access to behavioral health support and respite care options to reduce caregiver burnout and help families maintain emotional well-being. Partner with local community organizations to offer these services at reduced or no cost.
- **Resource Navigation Assistance**: Assign staff or volunteers to help families navigate community resources, such as financial assistance programs, local childcare options, and specialized therapies. This can alleviate stress and allow families to focus more on caregiving.
- **Cultural and Language-Specific Services**: Offer culturally sensitive support services that respect families' unique backgrounds, languages, and traditions. Provide interpreters, translated materials, and culturally adapted resources to make

information and services accessible to diverse populations.

5

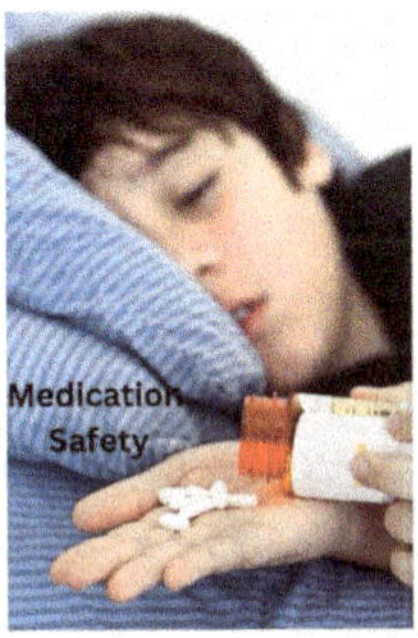

"Safe and Sound: Strategies for Preventing Medication Errors in Pediatric Healthcare"

Medication errors pose significant risks to pediatric patients and are a leading cause of adverse events in healthcare settings. In this chapter, we explore a comprehensive array of strategies for preventing medication errors in pediatric healthcare. By implementing robust protocols, enhancing communi-

CATION, AND PRIORITIZING PATIENT SAFETY, HEALTHCARE PROVIDERS can safeguard the well-being of pediatric patients and promote positive outcomes.

ROOT CAUSES OF MEDICAL ERRORS

Communication Failures

1. **Incomplete Information Transfer**: Miscommunication during handoffs or shift changes can lead to incomplete information transfer and subsequent errors.
2. **Lack of Standardization**: Inconsistent communication practices can result in misunderstandings and errors.

Human Factors

1. **Fatigue and Burnout**: Healthcare providers experiencing fatigue or burnout are more likely to make errors.
2. **Distraction and Multitasking**: Distractions and the need to multitask can lead to lapses in attention and mistakes.

Systemic Issues

1. **Inadequate Staffing**: Insufficient staffing levels can lead to increased workloads and a higher risk of errors.
2. **Lack of Resources**: Limited access to necessary resources, such as equipment or technology, can compromise patient safety.

MEDICATION ERRORS

Understanding the Scope of Medication Errors in Pediatrics

Prescribing, dispensing, and administering medications to pediatric patients involves unique challenges that can lead to higher risks of medication errors. Here's an in-depth look at these challenges and the factors contributing to potential errors:

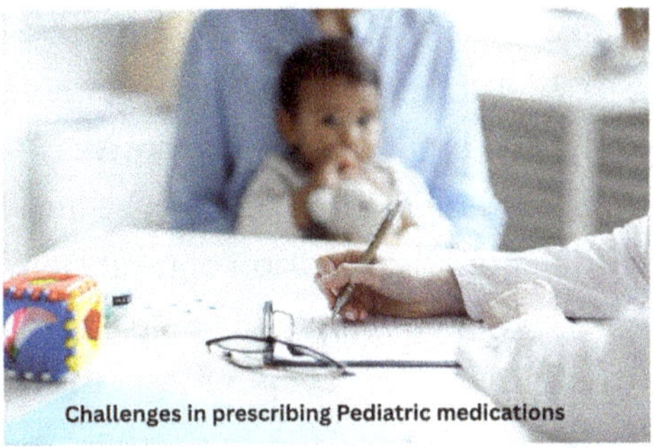

1. Unique Challenges in Prescribing Medications for Pediatric Patients

- **Age-Specific Dosage Calculations**: Pediatric patients range from neonates to adolescents, each with differing metabolic rates and body compositions. Unlike adults, pediatric dosing often depends on the child's weight or body surface area, making accurate dosing calculations complex and error-prone.
- **Limited Pediatric-Specific Formulations**: Many medications are primarily designed for adult use, which means that pediatric formulations or strengths are often unavailable. Providers may need to use off-label dosing or compounded medications, which increases the likelihood of dosing errors.
- **Variability in Pharmacokinetics and Pharmacodynamics**: Children metabolize and respond to medications differently due to ongoing physiological development. Factors like age, organ maturity, and enzyme activity influence drug absorption, distribution, metabolism, and excretion, making standardized dosing challenging.
- **Communication Limitations**: Young children may struggle to describe their symptoms or side effects accurately, making it harder for providers to gauge effectiveness or identify adverse reactions, leading to potential misinterpretation of treatment needs.

2. Unique Challenges in Dispensing Medications for Pediatric Patients

- **Specialized Compounding Requirements**: Pharmacists may need to prepare liquid or chewable formulations if tablets or capsules aren't appropriate for children. Compounding increases the risk of miscalculating dosages or introducing contaminants.

- **Lack of Standardized Dosing Devices**: Dispensing syringes, droppers, or cups may be inaccurately calibrated, leading to inconsistent dosing. Families may also use household measuring tools, which are often imprecise and contribute to dosing errors.
- **High-Risk Medications**: Certain medications, such as insulin, chemotherapy agents, and anticoagulants, have narrow therapeutic ranges, where even small errors in dispensing can cause severe adverse effects. Pediatric patients are particularly vulnerable to such errors due to their smaller body sizes and lower tolerance for overdose.

3. Unique Challenges in Administering Medications to Pediatric Patients

- **Difficulty in Swallowing Medication**: Many children, especially young ones, have difficulty swallowing pills or capsules, which may lead to improper dosing if the medication needs to be crushed, divided, or administered in liquid form.
- **Parental Administration Errors**: When medications are administered at home, parents or caregivers may inadvertently give incorrect doses or improperly administer the drug, particularly if they lack clear instructions or if the drug requires complex preparation.
- **Emotional Resistance from Patients**: Pediatric patients may resist taking medications, leading to challenges in administering accurate doses. In cases where children spit out, vomit,

or refuse medication, determining the exact dose absorbed is challenging, potentially leading to underdosing or overdosing.

- **High Sensitivity to Adverse Effects**: Due to their ongoing growth and development, pediatric patients can be more sensitive to medication side effects, and small dosing variations can lead to significant adverse reactions.

4. Factors Contributing to Medication Errors in Pediatric Patients

- **Calculation Errors**: Dosages based on weight or body surface area are prone to errors, especially if units are incorrectly converted or rounding adjustments are mishandled. Even a small calculation mistake can lead to substantial dosing inaccuracies.
- **Communication Gaps**: Miscommunication between providers, pharmacists, and caregivers can result in incorrect dosages or misunderstandings about how and when to administer the medication. In complex cases, multiple healthcare providers may be involved, increasing the risk of miscommunication.
- **Incomplete or Inaccurate Documentation**: Inaccurate or incomplete medical records, especially regarding a child's weight, allergies, or current medications, can lead to errors in prescribing and administering medication. Regular weight updates are critical for dosing but may be overlooked.
- **Lack of Pediatric-Specific Guidelines**: With limited pediatric-specific clinical trials and drug guidelines, many medications are prescribed off-label, leading to variations in dosing recommendations and potentially unsafe practices.

Inadequate Parent or Caregiver Training: Many caregivers are given little to no training on how to correctly measure and administer medication, which increases the risk of dosing errors. Without clear instructions and education, caregivers may misunderstand the frequency, timing, or dose required.

- **Complex Medication Regimens**: Pediatric patients with chronic or complex conditions may require multiple medications with different dosing schedules, increasing the likelihood of missed or duplicated doses. This can be overwhelming for both healthcare providers and families, making errors more likely.

Strategies to Mitigate Medication Errors in Pediatric Care

- **Standardized Weight-Based Dosing Charts**: Using standardized charts can reduce calculation errors by providing predetermined doses based on weight ranges. Integrating electronic dosing calculators in EMRs can also support accurate dosing.

- **Enhanced Communication Protocols**: Implementing clear communication protocols among healthcare teams and providing caregivers with detailed, easy-to-understand instructions can reduce misunderstandings and errors.

- **Parental and Caregiver Education Programs**: Educating families on the importance of accurate dosing, proper administration techniques, and using precise measuring tools is essential in reducing at-home errors. Also, parents should be advised against dividing medications into smaller doses or doubling doses without orders given by the prescribing provider because of family economic insufficiency.
- **Pharmacist Review and Counseling**: A Pharmacist's involvement in reviewing prescriptions and counseling families on proper administration methods can help catch and prevent dosing or dispensing errors.

- **Pediatric-Specific Medication Labels and Instructions**: Clear, pediatric-focused labeling, with age-appropriate dosing and administration instructions, can help families understand and follow medication protocols.

MEDICATION SAFETY PROTOCOLS

Enhancing Medication Safety Protocols

Effective medication safety protocols are essential for preventing errors in pediatric healthcare. Medication safety in pediatric care can be greatly enhanced by implementing best practices for medication reconciliation, standardized prescribing practices, and double-check procedures. Integrating technology, such as electronic prescribing systems and barcode medication administration, further strengthens these practices. Here's a breakdown of best practices and the role of technology:

1. Medication Reconciliation Best Practices

- **Thorough Medication History Review**: Obtain a complete and accurate history of the patient's current medications, including over-the-counter drugs, vitamins, and supplements. Involve parents or caregivers to capture information on any medications taken at home or prescribed by other providers.
- **Standardized Documentation**: Use structured forms or

electronic medical records (EMRs) to document medication names, dosages, routes, and frequencies. Ensure that information is standardized and clearly legible to all healthcare providers.

- **Reconciliation at Every Transition of Care**: Perform medication reconciliation whenever the patient transitions between different care settings (e.g., upon admission, discharge, or transfer within departments). This helps verify consistency in medications and prevents unintended omissions, duplications, or dosing errors.
- **Involve Multiple Team Members**: Encourage collaborative reconciliation by involving physicians, pharmacists, nurses, and caregivers. Each team member's unique perspective helps identify discrepancies and ensures comprehensive reviews.
- **Clear Communication with Families**: Educate families about any changes to their child's medication regimen. Provide written information and encourage questions to ensure families fully understand new prescriptions or discontinued medications.

2. Standardized Prescribing Practices

- **Use of Weight-Based Dosing Guidelines**: Establish guidelines for calculating doses based on weight or body surface area, which is critical in pediatric populations. Standardized dosing protocols help reduce errors related to miscalculation.
- **Utilize Pre-Approved Medication Formularies**: Limit prescribing to an established list of medications that have been thoroughly vetted for pediatric use, reducing off-label usage and potential adverse reactions.
- **Clear, Consistent Prescription Orders**: Avoid ambiguous abbreviations, such as "QD" for once daily or "U" for units, as these can be misinterpreted. Use plain language

and provide full instructions (e.g., "once daily in the morning").

• **Standardize Concentrations and Units**: Ensure that all medications are prescribed in the same units (e.g., mg/kg) to prevent errors in calculation or conversion. Avoid fractional doses if possible and always use metric measurements.

• **Automatic Alerts for Drug Interactions and Allergies**: Implement EMR alerts that warn prescribers of potential drug interactions, allergies, or dosing errors based on the child's weight or age. These alerts serve as a safeguard, helping providers make informed decisions.

3. Double-Check Procedures

• **Two-Person Verification for High-Risk Medications**: Require double-checks by two healthcare professionals for high-alert medications (e.g., chemotherapy, insulin, anticoagulants). Each individual independently reviews the dosage, route, and patient details before administration.

• **Independent Dose Calculation**: For weight-based dosing, two providers should independently calculate the dose and compare results. This double-check approach is particularly important in pediatrics, where small miscalculations can lead to significant errors.

• **Barcode Scanning**: Encourage the use of barcode scanning technology to verify the correct patient, medication, dose, route, and time. This process automates the check, helping prevent errors in real time.

• **Documentation of Double-Checks**: Document all double-checks in the patient's medical record, including the names of the healthcare providers involved, to create a clear accountability trail and provide a record for future reviews.

• **Family/Caregiver Verification**: Encourage caregivers to verify the medication, dosage, and timing whenever possible.

Educated families who feel empowered to ask questions can act as an additional layer of safety.

4. Role of Technology in Enhancing Medication Safety

• **Electronic Prescribing Systems (e-Prescribing)**

◦ **Automated Dose Calculation and Weight-Based Dosing**: e-Prescribing systems can automatically calculate weight-based doses, reducing errors caused by manual calculations

◦ **Clinical Decision Support (CDS) Alerts**: CDS embedded within e-prescribing systems can flag potential drug interactions, allergies, or dosing issues based on patient-specific factors such as age, weight, or other conditions.

◦ **Minimization of Illegible Prescriptions**: e-Prescribing eliminates the issue of handwriting legibility, ensuring that pharmacists and caregivers receive clear instructions.

◦ **Streamlined Communication with Pharmacies**: Electronic prescriptions are sent directly to pharmacies, reducing delays and transcription errors associated with faxing or handwritten prescriptions.

• **Barcode Medication Administration (BCMA)**

◦ **Right Patient Verification**: BCMA systems help confirm patient identity by scanning barcodes on the patient's wristband and matching it with the prescribed medication, reducing the chance of administering medication to the wrong patient.

◦ **Real-Time Dose Verification**: Scanning the medication's barcode ensures the correct dose is administered at the right time, enhancing adherence to dosing schedules and reducing the risk of missed doses or duplicate dosing.

Automated Documentation: BCMA systems automatically document each dose administered, creating an accurate, time-stamped record in the EMR. This helps providers track medication adherence and identify missed or delayed doses.

- **Automated Dispensing Cabinets (ADCs)**
  - **Controlled Access to Medications**: ADCs help prevent unauthorized access to medications and reduce errors by dispensing the exact dose needed based on the prescription order.
  - **Error Reduction in Medication Retrieval**: By organizing medications based on patient profiles, ADCs minimize retrieval errors, especially with look-alike or sound-alike drugs.
  - **Integration with EMRs**: ADCs can synchronize with EMRs, updating patient medication records in real-time and providing alerts if a drug is dispensed outside of the prescribed dose or frequency.
- **Telemedicine and Remote Monitoring**
  - **Access to Specialist Consultation**: Telemedicine enables quick access to pediatric specialists who can provide input on complex medication regimens, enhancing the accuracy of prescribing and administration.
  - **Real-Time Monitoring and Support**: Remote monitoring of medication adherence and side effects allows healthcare providers to respond promptly to issues, especially for high-risk patients or those with chronic conditions.

By implementing these best practices and leveraging technology, healthcare providers can enhance medication safety, minimize errors, and deliver safer, more effective care for pediatric patients.

Improving Medication Labeling and Packaging

Clear and accurate medication labeling and packaging are critical for preventing errors in pediatric medication administration. The strategies for improving medication labeling, include standardized formats, color-coded labels, and age-appropriate dosing instructions.

Improving medication labeling is essential to reducing errors and ensuring safe, accurate medication use in pediatric care. Here are strategies for enhancing medication labeling, as well as the importance of clear communication between health-care providers and pharmacists regarding medication orders.

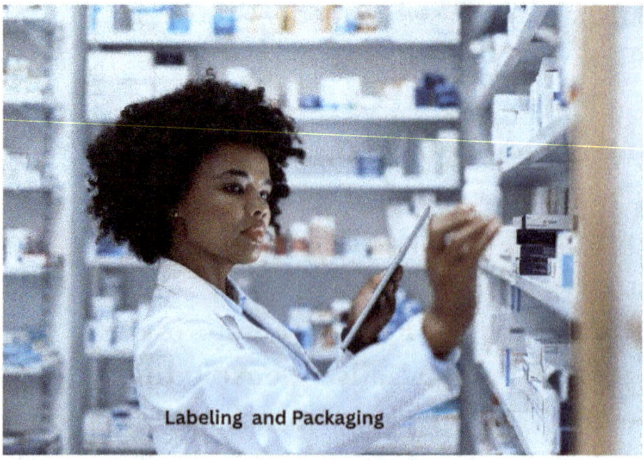

1. Standardized Label Formats

• **Consistent Layout and Terminology**: Use a standardized label format that includes essential information in a consistent order, such as the medication name, dose, frequency, route of administration, and expiration date. Avoid jargon or abbreviations that might confuse caregivers.

• **Bold and Clear Font**: Labels should use easy-to-read fonts and sizes, especially for critical information like dosage instructions. Bold or highlight the drug name and dose, as these are the most vital pieces of information.

• **Logical Grouping of Information**: Organize labels so that related information is grouped together. For instance, include dosing frequency and timing in the same area, and clearly separate warnings or contraindications.

Prominent Instructions for Storage and Safety: Labeling should include clear guidance on storage (e.g., refrigeration if required) and any safety precautions (e.g., "Keep out of reach of children").

2. Color-Coded Labels

• **Distinct Colors for High-Risk Medications**: Use specific colors to identify high-risk medications (e.g., red for anticoagulants or chemotherapy agents) to quickly alert caregivers and healthcare providers to exercise caution.

• **Color Coding by Administration Route**: Assign colors to represent different routes of administration, such as green for oral medications, blue for topical, and purple for injectables. This reduces the risk of administering medication via the wrong route.

• **Pediatric-Specific Color Coding**: Consider using color coding that indicates medications formulated or dosed specifically for pediatric use. This helps pharmacists and caregivers quickly identify child-appropriate medications.

3. Age-Appropriate Dosing Instructions

- **Weight-Based and Age-Based Dosage Charts**: Include dosing charts on the label or as an insert that clearly outlines dosing by age and weight categories. This is particularly important in pediatric patients, where dosing needs to be highly individualized.
- **Avoiding Fractions and Simplifying Measurements**: Whenever possible, avoid fractional doses (e.g., ½ teaspoon) to reduce dosing complexity. Use milliliter (mL) measurements and provide calibrated dosing devices (e.g., syringes or

droppers) to help caregivers accurately measure doses.

- **Clear Visuals and Simple Language**: Use graphics or icons for non-readers or caregivers who may struggle with medical terminology. Simple images indicating dose timing (e.g., morning, afternoon, bedtime) can also help.
- **Warning Labels for Age-Specific Restrictions**: If certain medications are contraindicated or pose specific risks for certain age groups, include clear warning labels that specify these age-based restrictions to prevent accidental administration.

4. The Importance of Clear Communication Between Healthcare Providers and Pharmacists

- **Clear, Consistent Terminology**: Standardize the language used between providers and pharmacists to minimize misunderstandings. Avoid using potentially ambiguous abbreviations or shorthand that could be misinterpreted (e.g., "U" for units, "QD" for once daily).
- **Verification of Dosing Calculations**: Encourage pharmacists to verify doses, especially in pediatric settings where weight-based dosing is required. Clear communication on patient age, weight, and health status allows pharmacists to double-check the dosing prescribed.
- **Collaborative Medication Reconciliation**: During transitions of care, ensure that providers and pharmacists work together to reconcile all medications, preventing duplications or omissions. This can reduce errors, particularly when patients

are moving between different departments or care settings.

- **Confirming Administration Instructions**: Providers should clearly convey any specific administration instructions (e.g., take with food, avoid certain foods or medications) to pharmacists. This ensures accurate labeling and clear guidance for families.
- **Streamlined Feedback Channels**: Establish systems (e.g., secure messaging within EMRs) that enable pharmacists to promptly ask questions or clarify ambiguities with prescribing providers. This open communication reduces errors and allows for real-time clarifications.
- Implementation of these strategies for labeling improvements and promoting clear, consistent communication between healthcare providers, pharmacists, and pediatric care teams can significantly enhance medication safety, reduce errors, and support families in accurately administering medications.

Educating Healthcare Providers and Families

Education is key to preventing medication errors in pediatric healthcare.

Comprehensive training for healthcare providers and effective education for families is crucial for ensuring medication safety in pediatric care. Here's why each is essential and the best strategies for achieving both.

Importance of Comprehensive Training for Healthcare Providers

1 Enhanced Patient Safety: Medication errors are a significant risk in pediatric care, where small miscalculations or incorrect doses can have severe consequences. Training providers on medication safety protocols build a culture of caution and precision, reducing the risk of harm.

2 Accurate Dosage Calculations: Pediatric dosing is often based on weight or body surface area, requiring precise calculations. Training reinforces the importance of accurate dose calculations and ensures providers are adept at using weight-based and age-specific dosing guidelines.

3 Understanding Pediatric Pharmacology: Children metabolize and respond to medications differently than adults. Specialized training in pediatric pharmacology helps providers understand these differences, ensuring they choose the correct medication and adjust doses based on developmental factors.

4 Confidence in High-Stakes Situations: When prescribing or administering high-risk medications (e.g., chemotherapy, insulin), providers must be well-versed in specific safety protocols. Regular training ensures healthcare providers can confidently manage these situations, reducing anxiety and enhancing focus on patient safety.

Training Strategies for Healthcare Providers

- **Regular Simulation-Based Training**: Use simulation scenarios that mimic real-life pediatric cases to help providers practice calculations, dosage adjustments, and medication administration. Simulations are particularly valuable for preparing providers for high-stakes situations in a controlled environment.
- **Standardized Protocol Education**: Ensure all providers are trained on standardized protocols for medication administration, double-checking procedures, and safety alerts. Regular reviews and

updates on protocols keep providers aligned with the latest best practices.

- **Pharmacology Workshops and Continuing Education**: Offer workshops and ongoing education on pediatric pharmacology, focusing on developmental factors influencing drug absorption, metabolism, and excretion. These sessions should also cover new research, updated guidelines, and emerging medications.
- **Cross-Disciplinary Case Reviews**: Encourage healthcare teams, including pharmacists, physicians, and nurses, to participate in regular case reviews focused on medication safety. These reviews allow for open discussions about complex cases, mistakes, and improvement strategies, promoting a culture of continuous learning and improvement.
- **Annual Competency Testing**: Implement annual testing to assess proficiency in medication safety protocols, dosage calculations, and pharmacology knowledge. Testing helps identify areas where providers may need additional training or support.

Educating Families on Safe Medication Administration

Educating families is essential, as they are often responsible for administering medications at home. Proper education reduces the risk of administration errors and increases adherence, which is vital for effective treatment.

Importance of Family Education

1 Empowered and Informed Caregivers: When families understand the medication, its purpose, and how to administer it correctly, they feel more confident in managing their child's care.

2 Reduction in Errors at Home: Families who are trained in administration techniques, dosage measurement, and timing are less likely to make mistakes, such as giving the wrong dose or frequency.

3 Early Detection of Side Effects: Educating families on potential side effects helps them recognize signs of adverse reactions early, allowing them to seek medical attention quickly.

4 Improved Adherence: When families understand the importance of medication adherence, they are more likely to follow the prescribed schedule, leading to better health outcomes for the child.

Strategies for Educating Families

- **Demonstration and Practice Sessions**: Before discharge or administering a new medication, provide hands-on training sessions where families can practice measuring and administering doses under the supervision of a healthcare provider. Offer dosing syringes, droppers, or other accurate measuring tools to reinforce the correct technique.
- **Easy-to-Understand Educational Materials**: Create materials with clear, step-by-step instructions, visuals, and simplified language. Include a dosing schedule, potential side effects to watch for, and contact information for questions. Consider video tutorials or app-based resources for added accessibility.
- **Teach-Back Method**: After providing education, ask families to explain or demonstrate what they learned. This approach confirms they understand the instructions and allows providers to clarify any misunderstandings.
- **Side Effect Awareness and Management Guidance**: Provide families with a list of common and serious side effects,

along with instructions on what to do if they notice any. Emphasize when to seek immediate medical attention, helping families feel more prepared and reducing the likelihood of delayed care.

- **Reinforce the Importance of Adherence**: Explain to families why adherence is crucial, particularly in chronic or critical conditions. Highlight the importance of timing, consistent dosing, and completing the course of medication even if symptoms improve.
- **Provide Contact Support**: Ensure families know how to reach healthcare providers if they have questions or concerns. Offering an on-call number or access to a pharmacist can be especially helpful for medication-related inquiries.

ERROR REPORTING

Promoting Interdisciplinary Collaboration

Interdisciplinary collaboration is essential for preventing medication errors and promoting patient safety in pediatric healthcare.

Effective communication and teamwork among healthcare providers, including physicians, nurses, pharmacists, and allied health professionals, are foundational to delivering safe, high-quality pediatric care. Collaborative care not only improves patient outcomes but also enhances satisfaction and reduces errors. Below are the key reasons why communication and teamwork are essential, along with strategies for fostering a culture of collaboration and accountability within healthcare teams.

Importance of Communication and Teamwork in Healthcare

1. **Enhanced Patient Safety**: Clear communication reduces the risk of medication errors, misdiagnoses, and gaps in care. When healthcare

providers consistently share critical patient information, it minimizes the chances of errors and ensures seamless continuity of care.

2. **Holistic Patient Care**: Teamwork allows for diverse perspectives from different specialties, enabling comprehensive care that addresses both the physical and emotional needs of patients and their families. Each team member contributes unique insights based on their specialized training, leading to more robust care plans.
3. **Improved Efficiency**: When healthcare providers work together effectively, they streamline processes, reduce redundancies, and manage resources efficiently. This allows for quicker decision-making, reduces patient wait times, and increases overall productivity in the healthcare setting.
4. **Increased Provider Satisfaction**: Collaborative environments support healthcare providers by promoting mutual respect and reducing the sense of isolation. A strong team culture can enhance job satisfaction, reduce burnout, and foster a sense of shared purpose among team members.
5. **Better Patient and Family Engagement**: Effective communication helps healthcare teams present a unified message to patients and families, building trust and encouraging active participation in the care process. Families are more likely to feel informed and empowered when they receive consistent information from the entire healthcare team.

Strategies for Fostering a Culture of Collaboration and Accountability

1. Establish Clear Roles and Responsibilities

• **Role Clarity**: Clearly define the roles and responsibilities of each team member to avoid confusion and overlap. By understanding each member's specific duties, healthcare teams can work more efficiently and avoid misunderstandings.

• **Role Flexibility**: While roles are defined, encourage flexibility to adapt to the needs of each case. Foster an environment where team members can step in to support each other when needed, especially in high-stress or time-sensitive situations.

• **Interdisciplinary Huddles and Meetings**: Regular interdisciplinary meetings allow each team member to share updates, clarify roles, and discuss each patient's care plan. This ensures everyone is aligned on goals and responsibilities.

2. Promote Open, Respectful Communication

• **Use Structured Communication Tools**: Tools like SBAR (Situation, Background, Assessment, Recommendation) help standardize communication, especially during handoffs, ensuring that critical information is conveyed concisely and accurately.

• **Encourage a Culture of Psychological Safety**: Create an environment where team members feel safe to speak up, ask questions, and express concerns. When individuals feel respected and valued, they are more likely to share observations that could improve patient outcomes.

• **Regular Feedback and Debriefing**: Encourage open feedback channels where team members can reflect on what worked well and identify areas for improvement. Post-shift debriefings or case reviews provide constructive opportunities to discuss challenges and foster mutual respect.

3. Implement Collaborative Decision-Making Processes

• **Interdisciplinary Rounds**: Hold daily or weekly rounds

that include input from all relevant healthcare providers, from physicians and nurses to pharmacists and social workers. This collaborative approach allows for well-rounded care plans that consider all aspects of the patient's health.

- **Joint Goal-Setting**: Involve the entire care team in setting short- and long-term goals for the patient. Collaborative goal-setting ensures that all providers are working toward the same outcomes and helps prevent conflicting or redundant interventions.
- **Shared Decision-Making with Families**: Engage families as part of the team by involving them in care discussions and decision-making processes. This approach enhances family trust and encourages open dialogue, especially regarding the patient's needs and values.

4. Utilize Technology to Support Teamwork

- **Electronic Health Records (EHR) for Unified Communication**: Use EHR systems that allow all providers involved in the patient's care to access and update records in real time. Unified EHR access minimizes communication gaps, providing up-to-date information on the patient's status and treatment.
- **Communication Platforms for Instant Updates**: Use secure communication platforms or apps that enable quick, real-time updates among team members. These tools are particularly useful for urgent situations or for sharing changes in care plans.
- **Shared Task Management Tools**: Implement task management systems that outline each team member's responsibilities and progress. This can enhance accountability and help prevent tasks from being missed.

5. Foster Accountability Through Clear Standards and Continuous Improvement

Set Shared Standards of Care: Develop standardized

protocols and guidelines that all team members follow, ensuring consistency and a shared commitment to high-quality care. Standards also provide a foundation for accountability, as each provider knows the benchmarks they are expected to meet.

Encourage Peer Accountability: Cultivate a culture where team members feel comfortable holding each other accountable in a constructive, supportive manner. This mutual responsibility reinforces shared goals and enhances teamwork.

- **Ongoing Training in Team-Based Care**: Offer training programs that emphasize the principles of teamwork, communication, and shared accountability. This can include workshops on team-building, leadership skills, and conflict resolution, which equip team members to handle challenging situations effectively.
- **Regular Performance Review and Quality Improvement Initiatives**: Evaluate team performance regularly through audits, feedback surveys, and case reviews. Use these assessments to identify areas for improvement, reward high-performing teams, and make any necessary adjustments to protocols or communication practices.

By prioritizing open communication, establishing clear standards, and embracing a team-based approach to care, healthcare providers can create an environment where collaboration and accountability thrive. This collaborative culture not only enhances the quality of care for pediatric patients but also promotes a supportive work environment, where all team members can contribute to and take pride in delivering the best possible care.

Implementing Error Reporting and Quality Improvement Initiatives

Error reporting systems and quality improvement initiatives are essential for identifying and addressing medication errors in pediatric healthcare.

Establishing robust reporting mechanisms, conducting root cause analyses, and implementing corrective actions are critical components of a proactive approach to patient safety. Together, these practices help healthcare organizations identify, address, and prevent the recurrence of errors, ultimately fostering a safer and more effective care environment.

1. Importance of Robust Reporting Mechanisms

- **Identification of Safety Issues**: A structured reporting mechanism encourages healthcare providers to document and report any incidents, near-misses, or potential safety concerns. This process allows organizations to identify patterns and vulnerabilities in the care process that could otherwise go unnoticed.
- **Fostering a Culture of Transparency**: Reporting systems promote openness by providing a non-punitive means for healthcare staff to share information about errors or near-misses. This transparency builds trust within the team and encourages staff to prioritize safety without fear of blame.
- **Timely Response and Mitigation**: With a robust reporting system in place, healthcare organizations can respond quickly to errors or potential hazards. Immediate action can mitigate the potential impact on patients, allowing teams to address and correct issues before they escalate.

2. Conducting Root Cause Analyses (RCAs)

Understanding the True Cause of Errors: RCAs delve into the underlying factors contributing to an error, going beyond surface-level symptoms to identify systemic issues that may have caused or contributed to the incident. This process is crucial for understanding the root causes rather than just addressing symptoms.

- **Identifying Systemic Issues and Preventative**

Measures: RCAs examine the error from multiple angles, considering human factors, procedural weaknesses, and environmental issues. By thoroughly investigating each factor, RCAs can uncover systemic issues, like communication breakdowns or procedural flaws, that might otherwise remain unaddressed.

- **Promoting a Blame-Free Culture**: RCAs focus on understanding processes and identifying points of improvement rather than assigning blame to individuals. This approach fosters a culture where healthcare providers feel safe discussing errors and working collaboratively to prevent recurrence, enhancing team cohesion and morale.

3. Implementing Corrective Actions

- **Transforming Insights into Actionable Solutions**: After identifying the root causes of an error, organizations need to implement corrective actions to prevent similar events in the future. These actions may involve revising protocols, enhancing training programs, or improving communication strategies. Corrective actions are a tangible demonstration of an organization's commitment to safety.
- **Continuous Monitoring and Adjustment**: Corrective actions are most effective when coupled with ongoing monitoring to ensure they're meeting their intended goals. Regular follow-up allows healthcare teams to adjust strategies as needed, ensuring that solutions remain relevant and effective over time.
- **Empowering Staff to Drive Improvement**: Implementing corrective actions creates opportunities for healthcare providers to be directly involved in quality improvement. When staff members see that their reports and insights lead to real change, they become more engaged and motivated to contribute actively to safety and quality initiatives.

Strategies for Building an Effective System of Reporting, Analysis, and Correction

1 Non-Punitive Reporting Policies: Encourage reporting by creating policies that protect individuals from disciplinary action when errors are reported in good faith. This helps reduce fear and ensures that all team members feel comfortable contributing to the organization's safety efforts.

2 Standardized Reporting Tools: Use standardized tools and processes (e.g., electronic incident reporting systems) that allow healthcare providers to report issues efficiently and accurately. User-friendly reporting systems streamline the process, encouraging higher reporting rates.

3 Cross-Functional RCA Teams: Establish RCA teams with diverse healthcare professionals, including physicians, nurses, pharmacists, and administrators. Cross-functional teams bring different perspectives to the analysis, leading to a more comprehensive understanding and solutions.

4 Transparent Communication of Findings and Actions: Share RCA findings and corrective actions with all relevant staff members. This transparency helps keep everyone informed, reinforces the importance of safety initiatives, and highlights the organization's commitment to continuous improvement.

5 Education and Training on Root Cause Analysis: Provide regular training on conducting RCAs, helping staff develop the skills to identify root causes and develop actionable solutions. This training empowers teams to apply RCA principles in their day-to-day work, promoting a more proactive approach to preventing errors.

Benefits of a Robust Reporting and RCA System

- **Reduced Error Recurrence**: By addressing the root causes and implementing corrective actions, healthcare organizations significantly reduce the likelihood of recurring errors, thereby enhancing patient safety.

- **Improved Trust and Morale Among Staff**: A well-implemented system shows staff that their concerns and contributions matter. This commitment to safety builds trust within the organization, strengthening morale and encouraging a proactive approach to patient care.
- **Enhanced Quality of Care and Patient Outcomes**: When healthcare providers feel safe reporting errors and participating in RCAs, the overall quality of care improves. Identifying and addressing weaknesses prevents adverse events and leads to better patient outcomes.

By establishing a robust framework for error reporting, root cause analysis, and corrective action, healthcare organizations create a continuous improvement cycle that promotes accountability and safety. This framework not only builds a culture of excellence but also ensures that every experience, including those involving errors, contributes to a safer, more effective healthcare environment for patients and providers alike.

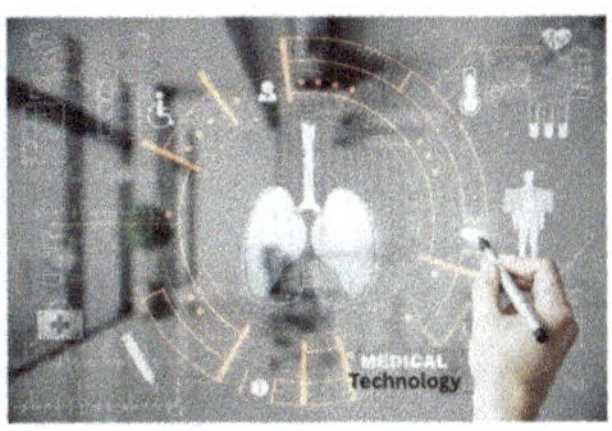

Embracing Technology and Innovation

Technology and innovation offer opportunities to enhance medication safety in pediatric healthcare.

Technology plays an increasingly critical role in preventing medication errors and ensuring safe medication practices. Innovations such as electronic health records, clinical decision support systems, and smart infusion pumps have revolutionized the ways healthcare providers manage medications, while emerging trends like tele-pharmacy services and artificial intelligence (AI) promise further improvements in medication safety.

Role of Key Technologies in Preventing Medication Errors

1 Electronic Health Records (EHRs)

- **Comprehensive Patient Information**: EHRs provide a complete, centralized record of a patient's medical history, including allergies, current medications, lab results, and diagnoses. This helps providers make informed decisions and reduces the risk of medication errors caused by incomplete information.
- **Automated Alerts and Flags**: EHRs include built-in alerts for potential medication interactions, duplicate therapies, or allergies, warning healthcare providers before an error occurs. These alerts are particularly valuable in high-volume environments where providers may be prone to oversight.
- **Standardization of Medication Orders**: EHRs help standardize medication orders by using structured templates and drop-down lists, reducing the likelihood of misinterpretations or dosing errors that might arise from handwritten prescriptions.

2 Clinical Decision Support Systems (CDSS)

- **Guided Decision-Making**: CDSSs are designed to assist providers by offering real-time, evidence-based recommendations during the prescribing and dispensing process. This includes dosing guidance tailored to the patient's age, weight, and kidney function, as well as suggested alternative medications if a drug interaction is detected.
- **Reducing Cognitive Load**: By automatically flagging

high-risk medications or complex dosing requirements, CDSSs alleviate some of the cognitive burden on healthcare providers, allowing them to focus on critical aspects of care rather than manually cross-checking for interactions or correct doses.

• **Integration with EHRs**: When integrated with EHRs, CDSSs enhance medication safety by using patient-specific data to guide decisions. For example, they can detect abnormal lab results that might contraindicate certain drugs or suggest dosage adjustments for high-risk patients.

1 Smart Infusion Pumps

◦ **Precise Dosing and Rate Control**: Smart infusion pumps are programmable devices that deliver medications intravenously with highly precise dosing controls. They help ensure that medications are administered at the correct rate and volume, particularly in cases requiring complex dosing, such as for neonates or patients on critical medications.

◦ **Built-In Drug Libraries and Safety Limits**: These pumps come equipped with drug libraries that include predefined safety limits for each medication, such as maximum and minimum infusion rates. If a nurse accidentally enters a dose outside these limits, the pump will automatically alert them, reducing the risk of over- or under-dosing.

◦ **Data Integration with EHRs**: Many smart infusion pumps can connect with EHRs to automatically document medication administration data, reducing manual data entry errors and ensuring accuracy in patient records.

Emerging Trends and Innovations in Medication Safety

1 Tele-pharmacy Services

◦ **Expanding Access to Pharmacist Expertise**: Tele-pharmacy services allow pharmacists to provide guidance remotely, ensuring that patients in underserved or rural areas have access to professional medication counseling. This increases adherence and reduces the chance of self-administered dosing errors.

- **Real-Time Medication Verification**: Through tele-pharmacy, pharmacists can review and verify prescriptions electronically, offering guidance to both patients and providers without the need for in-person consultations. This real-time verification helps prevent prescribing errors and provides timely support to healthcare teams.
- **24/7 Support for Complex Cases**: Tele-pharmacy services offer round-the-clock support, enabling healthcare providers to consult pharmacists for complex or high-risk cases at any time. This accessibility is particularly valuable for settings like emergency rooms and urgent care centers.

1 Artificial Intelligence (AI) in Medication Safety Artificial intelligence is revolutionizing healthcare—from improving surgical training and procedures to equipping healthcare providers with insights and personalizing care for patients around the world. Potential benefits of AI in healthcare include improving outcomes for both patients and clinical teams, lowering healthcare costs, and benefitting population health.[11]

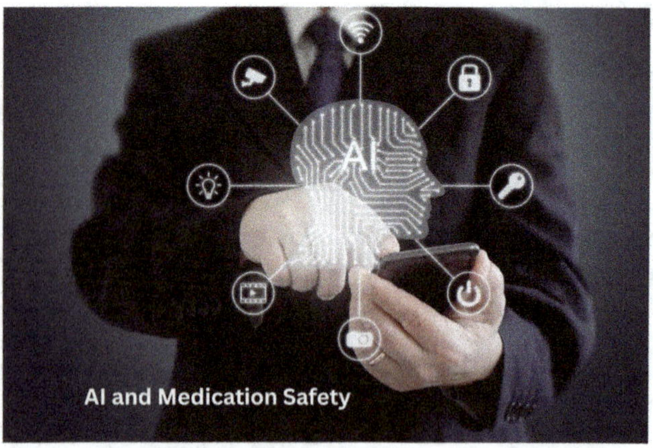

• **Predictive Analytics for Adverse Events**: AI algorithms can analyze large volumes of patient data to predict which patients are at a higher risk for adverse drug reactions. This helps providers take preventive measures, such as adjusting doses or choosing alternative treatments, before a negative event occurs.

• **Medication Reconciliation Automation**: AI-powered tools can assist with medication reconciliation by cross-referencing patient records, previous prescriptions, and current medications. This automation reduces the workload for providers and minimizes the risk of medication duplications or omissions.

• **Error Detection and Prescription Verification**: AI can rapidly analyze prescription orders, looking for inconsistencies or potential errors that may be missed by human providers. Some AI systems can even "learn" from past errors, continuously improving their accuracy in identifying risky orders.

Voice Recognition and Natural Language Processing (NLP):

NLP technology in AI systems can interpret free-text notes in EHRs and detect potential issues, such as conflicting medications or missed contraindications. This capability enhances the accuracy of medication orders, especially for complex cases or when providers use unstructured notes.

1 Blockchain for Secure Medication Tracking

◦ **Enhanced Traceability**: Blockchain technology offers secure tracking of medications from manufacturer to patient. This can be especially useful in preventing counterfeit medications and verifying the authenticity of drugs, particularly in high-stakes medications such as vaccines or controlled substances.

◦ **Immutable Records**: By maintaining an unalterable

record of medication transactions, blockchain technology can reduce errors and improve accountability within the supply chain. It enables better tracking of recalled medications and helps providers quickly respond to safety alerts.

2 Mobile Health (mHealth) and Medication Adherence Apps

- **Personalized Medication Reminders**: mHealth apps help patients adhere to their medication schedules by sending reminders and tracking missed doses. This is particularly helpful in chronic conditions, where long-term adherence is crucial to treatment success.
- **Interactive Features for Education**: Some mHealth apps provide patients with educational resources about their medications, potential side effects, and the importance of adherence. These interactive features help patients feel more engaged and empowered in managing their medications.

Conclusion

Technological advancements have significantly enhanced medication safety by reducing the likelihood of errors, streamlining complex processes, and supporting providers with real-time guidance. Established technologies like EHRs, CDSSs, and smart infusion pumps continue to be foundational in medication error prevention, while emerging tools like tele-pharmacy services, AI-driven systems, and blockchain offer exciting new possibilities for advancing patient safety. These innovations, combined with a proactive approach to adopting technology in healthcare, ensure that medication management becomes increasingly precise, safe, and accessible for all patients.

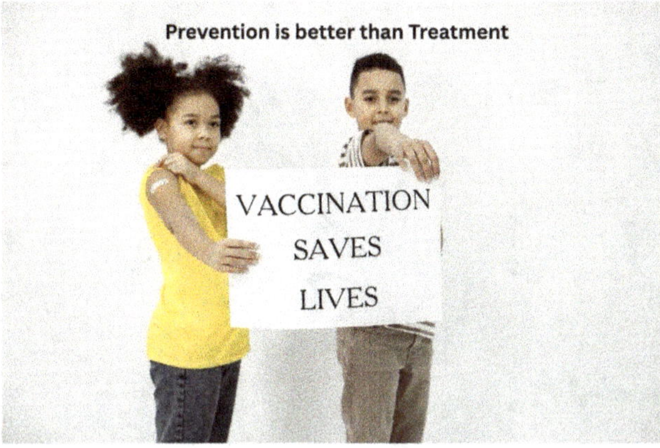
Prevention is better than Treatment
VACCINATION
SAVES
LIVES

6

TO VACCINATE OR NOT TO VACCINATE?

"Empowering Parents: Respecting Vaccine Hesitancy and Promoting Prevention of Vaccine-Preventable Diseases"

Vaccination is one of the most effective public health interventions, preventing millions of deaths and illnesses worldwide. However, vaccine hesitancy—defined as the delay in acceptance or refusal of vaccines despite the availability of vaccination services—poses a significant challenge to global immunization efforts.

Some vaccine-preventable diseases, like pertussis (whooping cough), chickenpox, and COVID-19, remain common in the United States. However, many other diseases, such as polio and diphtheria, are almost forgotten thanks to vaccines. If we stopped vaccinating, the few cases we have in the United States could very quickly become tens or hundreds of thousands of cases. Children who don't receive all vaccinations and are exposed to a disease can become seriously sick and spread it through a community.[12]

Understanding Vaccine Hesitancy

Vaccine hesitancy among parents is a multifaceted issue influenced by various factors, including concerns about vaccine safety and efficacy, distrust in healthcare providers, and widespread misinformation, particularly through social media.

Understanding these factors and the reasons behind parental hesitation or refusal to vaccinate their children is essential for healthcare providers, public health professionals, and policymakers who aim to improve vaccination rates and protect public health.

1. Concerns About Vaccine Safety and Efficacy

- **Fear of Side Effects**: One of the most common concerns among vaccine-hesitant parents is the potential for adverse side effects, especially rare but severe reactions. Some parents worry that vaccines could harm their children, potentially causing allergies, autoimmune conditions, or developmental issues.
    - **Perceived Risk vs. Benefit**: Parents sometimes question the necessity of vaccines, especially for diseases they perceive as low-risk or no longer common. For example, the success of vaccines has led to a decrease in diseases like measles and polio, making the threat feel distant and abstract. Without experiencing these illnesses firsthand, some parents may believe that the risks of vaccination outweigh the benefits. Case studies on the resurgence of measles in unvaccinated communities highlight the consequences of low vaccination rates and the real-world importance of immunization.

- **Doubts About Vaccine Efficacy**: Concerns about whether vaccines will work as intended also contribute to hesitancy. Some parents might point to cases where vaccinated individuals contract the disease (albeit often with milder symptoms) as evidence that vaccines are not fully effective, casting doubt on the value of immunization.

1. **Distrust in Healthcare Providers and Institutions**

- **Historical and Systemic Trust Issues**: Certain communities have historical reasons for distrust in medical institutions, often rooted in unethical practices and neglect, such as the Tuskegee Syphilis Study. Starting in 1932, 600 African American men from Macon County, Alabama, were enlisted to partake in a scientific experiment on syphilis. The "Tuskegee Study of Untreated Syphilis in the Negro Male" was conducted by the United States Public Health Service (USPHS) and involved blood tests, x-rays, spinal taps, and autopsies of the subjects. The goal was to "observe the natural history of untreated syphilis" in black populations. However, the subjects were unaware of this and were simply told they were receiving treatment for bad blood. They received no treatment at all. Even after penicillin was discovered as a safe and reliable cure for syphilis, the majority of men did not receive it.[13] These histories can make parents wary of public health recommendations, including vaccines.
- **Transparency and Communication**: Parents may feel that they don't receive adequate information

from healthcare providers, or they may perceive that vaccine information is one-sided or dismissive of their concerns. If parents feel their questions are not taken seriously, they may turn to alternative sources for information or develop further skepticism.

- **Concerns About Pharmaceutical Industry Influence**: Some parents distrust the pharmaceutical industry, viewing it as motivated primarily by profit rather than public health. This perception can create doubt about the intentions behind vaccine recommendations and fuel suspicions about potential conflicts of interest among healthcare providers or regulatory agencies.

3. Misinformation Spread Through Social Media and the Internet

- **Access to Misinformation**: Social media platforms and websites provide access to vast amounts of information, some of which is inaccurate or misleading. Misinformation can appear compelling, particularly when shared by friends or individuals who seem credible. These messages often use emotional appeals or anecdotal evidence to stir fear, making them persuasive to concerned parents.

- **Echo Chambers and Confirmation Bias**: Online algorithms often create echo chambers by promoting content aligned with users' preexisting beliefs. Parents who have concerns about vaccines may unintentionally find themselves in online communities that reinforce those doubts, fueling vaccine hesitancy further.

- **Celebrity and Influencer Influence**: Some public figures, influencers, or celebrities express skepticism toward vaccines, which can lead parents to question vaccine safety and efficacy. When trusted voices raise doubts, they can hold significant sway over followers who view them as role models or sources of information.

4. Complex Personal Beliefs and Philosophical Concerns

- **Desire for "Natural" Immunity**: Some parents believe that natural immunity—acquired by contracting and recovering from a disease—is superior to vaccine-induced immunity. This perspective may stem from a preference for holistic or natural health practices, leading some to view vaccines as an artificial intervention.

- **Autonomy and Freedom of Choice**: Parents who value autonomy may resist vaccine mandates or feel uneasy about what they perceive as pressure from healthcare systems. This can be exacerbated when mandates are in place for school entry or employment, as some parents feel this infringes on their rights to make personal medical decisions for their children.
- **Personal or Cultural Beliefs**: In some cases, religious or philosophical beliefs influence a parent's decision. Certain religious groups oppose

vaccination, while other parents may hold personal convictions that emphasize individual choice over community responsibility.

5. Lack of Trust in Scientific Research and Regulatory Processes

- **Concerns About New Vaccines**: When new vaccines are introduced, especially during public health emergencies (e.g., COVID-19), some parents may be concerned about the rapid development process and perceive that safety testing is insufficient. This is often rooted in a misunderstanding of the accelerated regulatory processes, which are designed to maintain rigorous safety standards.

- **Skepticism Toward Vaccine Approval and Regulation**: Some parents worry that government regulatory bodies may be influenced by pharmaceutical interests or may not be as transparent as they should be. This skepticism extends to concerns that vaccine data could be manipulated or that long-term side effects might be hidden.

Addressing Vaccine Hesitancy: A Collaborative Approach

- **Improved Communication from Healthcare Providers**: Providers can help build trust by using empathy, listening to parents' concerns, and providing clear, evidence-based information about vaccine safety and efficacy. Open conversations that address parents' concerns, rather than one-size-fits-all messaging, can foster trust and facilitate informed decision-making.

- **Combating Misinformation with Accurate Information**: Public health agencies and healthcare organizations can counter misinformation by providing
- accessible, engaging, and accurate information through social media, websites, and community outreach. Partnering with trusted figures within communities can also be effective.

Community-Based Education Programs: Education programs that are community-specific and culturally sensitive can address local concerns and correct misconceptions. Providing factual, approachable information in a non-judgmental manner is key to encouraging open dialogue.

- **Supporting Vaccine-Confident Peer Networks**: Peer networks or community leaders who share positive vaccine experiences can be influential in changing minds. These voices offer relatable perspectives and can help alleviate fears by sharing their own vaccination experiences.

Conclusion

Vaccine hesitancy is a complex issue driven by concerns about safety and efficacy, distrust in healthcare providers, and the spread of misinformation. Addressing vaccine hesitancy requires a multifaceted, empathetic approach that acknowledges parental concerns and focuses on building trust.

By addressing these factors with transparency, evidence-based information, and respect for individual beliefs, healthcare providers and public health professionals can work towards encouraging informed, confident decisions about vaccination.

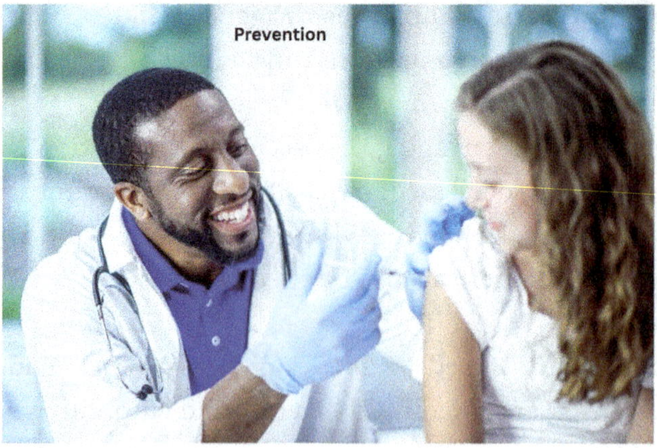

ADDRESSING VACCINE MISINFORMATION

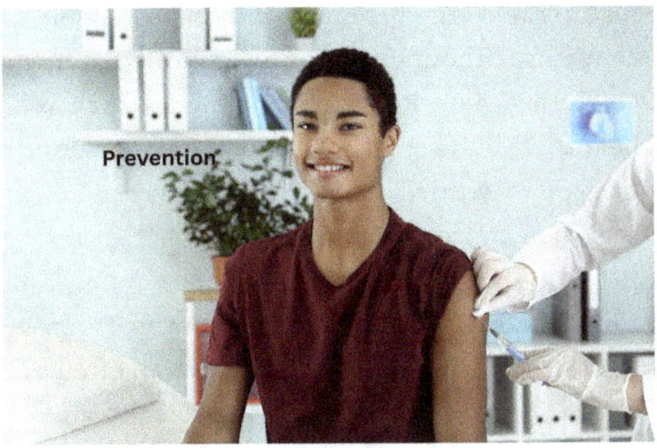

Addressing Vaccine Misinformation

Respectful communication is essential for addressing vaccine hesitancy and building trust with parents.

Engaging with vaccine-hesitant parents requires a respectful and empathetic approach that builds trust and fosters open dialogue. Rather than simply providing information, effective engagement involves active listening, acknowledging concerns, and delivering evidence-based information in a way that respects parents' autonomy and values. Addressing misinformation with empathy and clarity is also essential, as it empowers parents to make informed decisions for their children's health.

1. Active Listening and Empathy

- **Creating a Safe, Open Space**: Start conversations by ensuring that parents feel comfortable sharing their thoughts and concerns. Demonstrating genuine curiosity about their perspective can create a foundation of trust and signal that their input is valued.
- **Listening Without Interruptions**: Active listening requires allowing parents to fully express their concerns without interrupting or immediately correcting them. Reflective statements, such as "I hear that you're concerned about..." or "It sounds like you're worried about..." can reassure parents that their concerns are understood.

- **Empathizing with Parental Concerns**: Parents who hesitate to vaccinate their children often do so out of a deep desire to protect their health and well-being. Acknowledging these intentions—rather than focusing solely on the facts—can build rapport. Statements like, "I can understand why you'd want to make sure that everything is safe for your child," validate their concerns, making them more receptive to further discussion.

2. Acknowledging and Validating Concerns

- **Normalizing Worries About Safety**: Reassure parents that it is normal and responsible to be cautious about their children's health. Many parents may feel hesitant due to uncertainty or fear of judgment. Normalizing their questions by saying, "It's very common for parents to have concerns about this," can reduce any sense of isolation or defensiveness.
- **Identifying Shared Goals**: Emphasize the shared objective of keeping their child safe and healthy. Acknowledging a shared purpose helps position you as an ally rather than an authority figure, making parents more open to hearing new information.
- **Addressing Concerns Head-On**: Directly address specific fears or doubts, whether they're about potential side effects, vaccine ingredients, or the necessity of certain vaccines. Instead of dismissing these worries, provide a factual yet empathetic response. For example, if a parent is concerned about side effects, explain that while mild side effects are common, severe reactions are exceedingly rare and closely monitored.

3. Providing Evidence-Based Information in a Nonjudgmental Way

- **Communicating Facts Clearly and Simply**: Use simple, jargon-free language to explain how vaccines work, their safety, and why they are effective. Focusing on key messages, such as the role of vaccines in preventing serious illnesses, can help clarify complex information in a way that's accessible and reassuring.

- **Offering Data with a Personal Touch**: When possible, personalize the information to reflect the parent's situation, addressing concerns relevant to their child's age, health conditions, or family history. Sharing relatable stories, such as how other families in similar situations made decisions, can also make the information more relatable and less abstract.
- **Framing Information Positively**: Rather than focusing on what might happen if a child is not vaccinated, emphasize the benefits of vaccination, such as protecting their child from serious diseases and contributing to community health. Positive framing can make parents feel empowered and involved in a proactive health decision, rather than being pressured into a compliance-based choice.

4. Addressing Misinformation Respectfully

- **Correcting Misinformation with Empathy**: When misinformation arises, address it without judgment. Acknowledge the validity of the parent's concerns and provide correct information gently. For example, if a parent expresses fear of autism linked to vaccines, explain that extensive research has shown no link, reinforcing that scientific studies prioritize children's safety and well-being.
- **Referencing Trusted Sources**: Point parents to reputable sources, such as the Centers for Disease Control and Prevention (CDC) or the American Academy of Pediatrics (AAP), for additional

information. Suggesting sources respected by both the medical and public communities can strengthen your information and provide parents with credible places to continue their research.

- **Encouraging Critical Thinking**: Encourage parents to ask questions and critically evaluate sources. Explain how to identify reliable information, such as
- checking the credentials of sources and looking for scientific backing. Empowering them with tools to navigate misinformation helps them feel more in control and less dependent on conflicting online opinions.

5. Using Motivational Interviewing Techniques

- **Exploring Ambivalence**: Motivational interviewing is particularly useful in guiding vaccine-hesitant parents through their ambivalence without pressuring them into an immediate decision. Questions like "What are your biggest concerns about vaccines?" or "What would make you feel more comfortable?" allow parents to examine their thoughts and reveal potential paths to a resolution.
- **Eliciting "Change Talk"**: When parents express any positive statements about vaccines, such as "I want to protect my child from getting sick," reflect on these comments. This approach helps them reinforce their motivations and allows you to guide them toward weighing the pros and cons of vaccination in a supportive, non-directive manner.

- **Supporting Their Autonomy**: Rather than dictating a course of action, let parents feel they are part of the decision-making process. Phrases like, "I can provide all the information, but ultimately, the choice is yours," show respect for their autonomy and may lead them to consider vaccination more seriously.

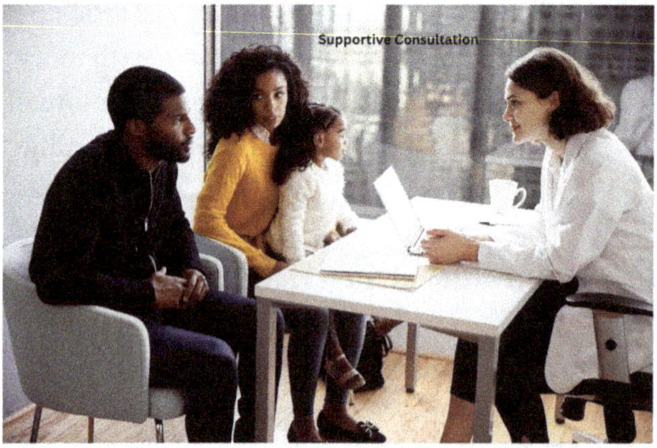

- **Building Relationships Over Time**: Vaccine hesitancy often cannot be resolved in a single conversation, especially if parents have deeply held beliefs. Approach each interaction as part of an ongoing relationship, showing consistent support and respect. By demonstrating that you're invested in the long-term well-being of their child, you increase the likelihood that they will eventually trust your guidance.
- **Offering Follow-Up Resources and Open Communication**: Provide pamphlets, links to trusted websites, or offer to revisit the conversation at a future appointment. Encouraging parents to

reach out with further questions lets them know that they have ongoing support and that vaccine-related discussions are welcome at any time.

Conclusion

Respectful, empathetic engagement with vaccine-hesitant parents can create a meaningful impact, guiding them toward informed, confident decisions. Strategies like active listening, validating concerns, and providing clear, evidence-based information can foster trust, while empathy and a nonjudgmental approach help parents feel respected and understood. Addressing misinformation gently, combined with motivational interviewing techniques, empowers parents to critically evaluate their options. Ultimately, consistent, respectful engagement supports a positive relationship between parents and healthcare providers, contributing to higher vaccination rates and healthier communities.

COMMON MYTHS

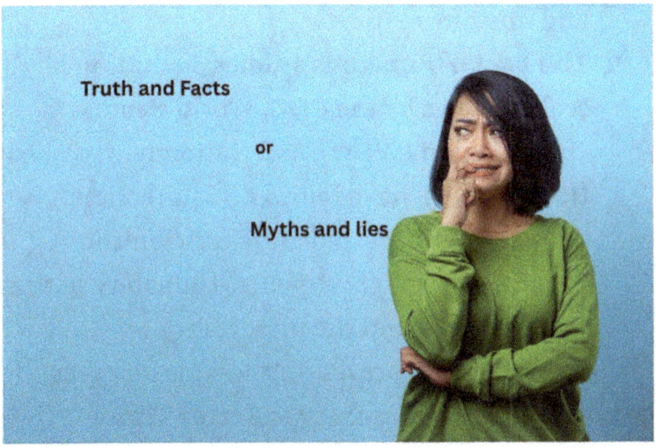

Misinformation and myths surrounding vaccines can fuel vaccine hesitancy and erode trust in immunization programs. Common myths and misconceptions about vaccines continue to drive vaccine hesitancy, fueled by misinformation and mistrust. Misconceptions range from concerns about vaccine ingredients to fears of long-term health effects. Effective strategies to debunk these myths involve a combination of education, transparency, and communication campaigns grounded in scientific evidence. Clear, empathetic messaging and accessible, trustworthy information can help counter these myths and foster vaccine confidence among parents and the public.

Common Myths and Misconceptions About Vaccines

1. **Myth: Vaccines Cause Autism**
    - **The Origin**: This misconception began with a now-debunked study published in the 1990s, which falsely linked the MMR (measles, mumps, rubella) vaccine to autism. Despite overwhelming evidence disproving the link, this myth persists, fueled by personal anecdotes and misinformation.
    - **The Facts**: Numerous studies, including large-scale reviews by the CDC, World Health Organization (WHO), and National Institutes of Health (NIH), have found no connection between vaccines and autism. Scientific consensus strongly supports the safety of the MMR vaccine and the importance of vaccination in preventing serious diseases.
2. **Myth: Natural Immunity Is Better Than Vaccine-Induced Immunity**
    - **The Origin**: Some people believe that recovering from an illness leads to stronger immunity than vaccination does, particularly for diseases like measles and chickenpox.

- **The Facts**: While natural infection can sometimes lead to immunity, it comes with significant risks. Contracting diseases like measles, polio, or COVID-

19 can cause serious, long-term complications or even death. Vaccines provide immunity safely, without exposing individuals to the disease's dangers.

3. **Myth: Vaccines Overload the Immune System**
    - **The Origin**: With several vaccines administered in early childhood, some parents worry that these will "overload" their child's immune system, causing harm or weakening it.
    - **The Facts**: Studies have shown that the immune system can handle the simultaneous introduction of multiple antigens (proteins in vaccines that stimulate immunity). Vaccines contain only a fraction of the antigens the immune system encounters daily from the environment. Additionally, vaccines are rigorously tested for safety to ensure they do not overwhelm the immune system.
4. **Myth: Vaccines Contain Harmful Ingredients, Such as Mercury**
    - **The Origin**: Concerns about vaccine ingredients, particularly thimerosal (a mercury-containing preservative), have led to fears that vaccines could be toxic.
    - **The Facts**: Thimerosal was removed from most vaccines as a precaution, despite evidence showing it to be safe in small amounts. It has never been in MMR vaccines, and today, the majority of vaccines for children contain no thimerosal. Other ingredients, like formaldehyde and aluminum, are present in trace amounts and have been proven safe.

Rigorous safety standards ensure that vaccine components are well within safe limits.

5. **Myth: COVID-19 Vaccines Were Developed Too Quickly to Be Safe**
    - **The Origin**: The rapid development and rollout of COVID-19 vaccines have raised safety concerns, with some fearing that the vaccines skipped important testing steps.
    - **The Facts**: COVID-19 vaccines went through all standard safety and efficacy trials, with unprecedented resources and collaboration that accelerated development. These vaccines underwent extensive testing with tens of thousands of participants, meeting regulatory standards worldwide. Continuous monitoring confirms their safety and effectiveness.

STRATEGIES FOR DEBUNKING MISINFORMATION

3. Education Through Evidence-Based Information

- **Providing Accessible Scientific Explanations**: Understandably, presenting science is key to addressing vaccine misconceptions. Healthcare providers and public health campaigns should use easy-to-grasp analogies, infographics, and videos to explain complex scientific concepts.
- **Tailoring Information to Different Audiences**: Educational efforts should cater to diverse audiences. Parents, teachers, healthcare workers, and young adults may have different concerns and access to information. Tailoring resources to these groups can make messages more effective.
- **Building Vaccine Literacy in Schools**: Incorporating basic information about vaccines into school curricula helps younger generations understand their importance. Teaching vaccine

science, the immune system, and public health principles fosters a foundation of trust and knowledge from an early age.

4.Transparency About Vaccine Safety and Development

- **Explaining the Vaccine Development Process**: Clear information on the steps involved in vaccine testing, development, and approval—along with post-market monitoring—can reassure the public. Showing the layers of oversight involved in vaccine approval processes helps reinforce their rigor and reliability.
- **Addressing Side Effects Honestly**: Being transparent about potential side effects, even minor ones, can improve trust. When healthcare providers or public health materials openly acknowledge possible side effects, it reduces fear and clarifies that these risks are minor and typically short-lived.
- **Data and Case Studies**: Sharing statistics on vaccine safety alongside real-world stories of individuals affected by vaccine-preventable diseases can be powerful.

5. Communication Campaigns Grounded in Empathy and Scientific Evidence

- **Developing Positive, Consistent Messaging**: Campaigns that highlight the positive impact of vaccines, such as protecting family and community, create a sense of shared purpose.

Simple, powerful slogans like "Vaccines Protect Us All" focus on community benefits and collective responsibility.

- **Utilizing Trusted Community Leaders and Voices**: Partnering with community influencers, religious leaders, or local figures who can resonate with different demographics makes vaccine campaigns more relatable. Trusted messengers within a community can help counter misinformation by offering reliable perspectives.
- **Storytelling and Testimonials**: Personal stories from parents who chose to vaccinate or who experienced the positive effects of immunization help counteract fear-based misinformation. Testimonials from healthcare workers, who witness the impact of vaccines and the consequences of vaccine-preventable illnesses firsthand, are also effective.

6. Addressing Misinformation on Social Media

- **Quickly Responding to Misinformation**: Public health agencies can monitor social media for misinformation and respond with factual posts. Correcting misinformation promptly, with respectful language, can prevent it from spreading.
- **Working with Social Media Platforms**: Social media companies increasingly collaborate with health organizations to limit the spread of harmful misinformation. Platforms can promote verified content on vaccine safety and health information in partnership with reliable sources, like the WHO or CDC.

- **Educational Campaigns in Digital Spaces**: Digital campaigns that promote "fact-checking" tools, direct readers to reliable resources, or link to public health websites are essential. These efforts empower users to verify information and encourage healthy skepticism toward sensationalized or unverified vaccine claims.

7. Empowering Healthcare Providers to Communicate Effectively

- **Training in Empathetic Communication**: Healthcare providers should be trained to approach vaccine discussions with empathy and openness, especially when talking to vaccine-hesitant parents. Rather than lecturing or dismissing concerns, providers can validate parental worries and offer evidence-based information in a way that builds trust.
- **Addressing Individual Concerns**: Providers should listen to each parent's specific worries and tailor their responses accordingly. Taking time to explain and answer questions—rather than simply promoting vaccines—can make parents feel heard and respected.

Conclusion

Debunking vaccine myths requires education, transparency, and targeted communication campaigns rooted in scientific evidence. By using clear explanations, transparent information about vaccine safety, and empathy-based communication strategies, healthcare providers and public health organizations can counteract misinformation and foster trust in vaccines. Building vaccine confidence is an ongoing effort that hinges on community engagement, respectful dialogue, and a commitment to accessible, evidence-based information. Through these strategies, we can combat misinformation and support informed decisions that contribute to public health and well-being.

BENEFITS OF VACCINATION

1. **Benefits of Vaccination**

Vaccination has long been a cornerstone of public health, offering multiple benefits not only to individuals but also to communities at large:

- Prevention of Disease: Vaccines prevent the onset of various infectious diseases, including measles, polio, influenza, and more, often reducing or eradicating disease in specific regions.
- Herd Immunity: Widespread immunization protects individuals who may be unable to get vaccinated due to age, health conditions, or other factors by reducing the overall presence of disease in the community.
- Reduction of Health Care Costs: Vaccines help reduce healthcare costs by preventing diseases that require costly treatments and hospitalizations.
- Prevention of Long-Term Complications: Vaccination can prevent diseases that may lead to

long-term health complications, helping people live healthier lives and avoiding disabilities associated with certain infections.

- Protection of Future Generations: Immunization programs help protect future generations, as vaccinated mothers and the reduced presence of diseases in communities reduce the likelihood of disease transmission to infants and children.

2. **Safety and Efficacy of Vaccines**

Vaccines are held to rigorous standards to ensure their safety and efficacy through multi-phase trials and ongoing monitoring:

- Rigorous Testing: Before approval, vaccines undergo several phases of clinical trials. Phase I focuses on safety, Phase II on efficacy and dosing, and Phase III on large-scale effectiveness and side effects across a diverse population.
- Continuous Monitoring: Even after a vaccine is approved, its safety and efficacy are continuously monitored through systems like the Vaccine Adverse Event Reporting System (VAERS) and the Vaccine Safety Datalink (VSD). This helps quickly identify and address any rare or long-term adverse effects.
- Transparency and Public Review: Agencies like the FDA and CDC regularly publish safety and efficacy data, enabling public scrutiny and fostering trust in the vaccine development process.
- Adaptation to New Variants: Vaccines, particularly for viruses that mutate quickly (e.g., influenza,

COVID-19), are periodically reviewed and adapted to remain effective against evolving variants.

EMPOWERING PARENTS TO BECOME ADVOCATES

3. **Strategies for Empowering Parents to Become Advocates for Vaccination**

Empowering parents as advocates within their communities can strengthen public confidence and promote vaccine uptake:

- Educational Programs: Providing parents with easy access to reliable, science-backed information on vaccine benefits and safety can empower them to confidently discuss vaccines with others.
- Encouraging Personal Testimonies: Sharing personal stories of positive vaccination experiences can resonate with other parents, deciding to vaccinate feels more relatable and trustworthy.
- Community Engagement: Holding Q&A sessions or forums with healthcare professionals allows parents to address their concerns and ask questions, helping them become informed, active advocates.

- Support from Pediatricians and Trusted Figures: Pediatricians and local leaders play a critical role in educating parents. By working closely with these trusted figures, parents can receive direct, credible guidance.

4. **Addressing Disparities in Vaccine Access and Equity**

Underserved communities often face barriers to vaccination that can lead to preventable outbreaks and health disparities. Addressing these inequities is crucial:

- Barriers to Vaccine Access: Common barriers include limited access to healthcare facilities, financial and logistical challenges, lack of information, and, in some cases, mistrust in healthcare due to historical inequities.
- Targeted Outreach: Establishing vaccination sites in easily accessible locations such as schools, community centers, and places of worship can make vaccinations more reachable. Mobile clinics are another effective strategy, particularly for rural areas.
- Community Engagement: Engaging community leaders and members in the vaccine rollout process can improve trust and increase vaccine uptake. Culturally tailored communications that resonate with specific community values and experiences can also help address hesitancy.

- Partnerships with Trusted Organizations: Partnering with trusted community organizations, such as local non-profits and advocacy groups, enables healthcare providers to connect with underserved populations in a familiar, trusted setting. These organizations can facilitate information dissemination, helping ensure that messages about vaccine safety and access reach everyone in the community.

Ensuring equitable access to vaccines and supporting informed decision-making through education and advocacy are vital to maintaining community health and achieving widespread immunity. Together, these efforts can help overcome barriers, reduce disparities, and build a healthier, well-protected future for all.

Respecting parental vaccine hesitancy while promoting the prevention of vaccine-preventable diseases requires a multifaceted approach grounded in empathy, education, and community engagement. By understanding parents' concerns, addressing misinformation, and highlighting the benefits of vaccination, healthcare providers and public health advocates can foster trust, promote vaccine acceptance, and protect the health of children and communities worldwide.

Let the goal be to provide healthcare providers, public health professionals, and community advocates with a comprehensive guide to respecting parental vaccine hesitancy while promoting vaccination as a critical tool for preventing vaccine-preventable diseases. Through respectful communication, education, and collaboration, we can empower parents to make informed decisions about vaccination and ensure that all children have access to the lifesaving benefits of immunization.

7

SHARED-DECISION MAKING BY PARENTS

Shared Decision-Making (SDM) by Parents in Pediatric Care

In pediatric care, decision-making is a dynamic and complex process that involves the child, parents or guardians, and healthcare professionals. Shared decision-making (SDM) is an approach that ensures that all parties participate in the healthcare decisions that affect the child. This process is fundamental to delivering high-quality, patient-centered care.

The principles, benefits, and challenges of SDM in pediatric care provide best practices for healthcare providers to facilitate effective shared decision-making.

Principles of Shared Decision-Making

Shared decision-making is rooted in the principles of autonomy, beneficence, non-maleficence, and justice. In pediatric care, these principles must be adapted to account for the developmental stages and legal dependency of children.

Key principles of SDM include:

1. **Collaboration**: Decisions are made jointly by healthcare

providers and parents, with consideration given to the child's views and preferences.

2. **Informed Choice**: Parents are provided with comprehensive, unbiased information about treatment options, including potential benefits, risks, and uncertainties.

3. **Respect for Preferences**: The values, preferences, and cultural beliefs of the family are respected and integrated into the decision-making process.

4. **Child-Centered Focus**: The child's best interests are the primary concern, and their evolving capacity to participate in decisions is acknowledged and supported.

The Role of Parents in Decision-Making

Parents or guardians are the primary decision-makers for their children's health care. Their role involves:

1. **Advocacy**: Acting in the best interests of the child by advocating for appropriate care and services.

2. **Interpreter**: Understanding and translating medical information to make informed choices.

3. **Emotional Support**: Providing emotional stability and reassurance to the child during the decision-making process.

4. **Ethical Steward**: Ensuring that decisions align with ethical considerations, including the child's quality of life and future well-being.

Benefits of Shared Decision-Making

Implementing SDM in pediatric care has numerous benefits:

1. **Improved Health Outcomes**: Collaborative decisions often lead to better adherence to treatment plans and improved health outcomes.

2. **Enhanced Satisfaction**: Parents who are actively involved in decision-making report higher satisfaction with care.

3. **Empowerment**: SDM empowers parents by valuing their insights and expertise regarding their child's needs.

4. **Trust Building**: It fosters trust between healthcare providers and families, which is crucial for effective healthcare delivery.

Challenges in Shared Decision-Making

Despite its benefits, SDM in pediatric care faces several challenges:

1. **Complexity of Information**: Medical information can be complex and difficult for parents to understand, especially in high-stress situations.

2. **Emotional Stress**: The emotional burden of making significant health decisions for a child can be overwhelming.

3. **Differing Perspectives**: Conflicts may arise between parents' wishes, the child's preferences, and medical recommendations.

4. **Time Constraints**: SDM can be time-consuming, which can be challenging in busy clinical settings.

Best Practices for Healthcare Providers in SDM:

To effectively facilitate SDM in pediatric care, healthcare providers can adopt the following best practices:

1. **Effective Communication**: Use clear, jargon-free language and visual aids to explain medical conditions and treatment options. Verify understanding through teach-back methods.

2. **Active Listening**: Practice active listening to understand parents' concerns, values, and preferences fully.

3. **Empathy and Support**: Provide empathetic support to parents, acknowledging the emotional difficulty of decision-making.

4. **Incorporate the Child's Voice**: Engage the child in the

decision-making process appropriate to their developmental level, ensuring their voice is heard and considered.

5. **Structured Frameworks**: Utilize decision aids and structured frameworks to help organize information and guide discussions.

6. **Collaborative Approach:** Foster a collaborative atmosphere where all team members, including nurses, social workers, and specialists, support the SDM process.

7. **Ongoing Education:** Educate families continuously, not just at the point of decision-making, to build their knowledge and confidence over time.

Shared decision-making is essential in pediatric care, ensuring that healthcare decisions reflect the best interests of the child while respecting the values and preferences of the family. By adopting best practices in SDM, healthcare providers can enhance patient outcomes, improve satisfaction, and build stronger, trust-based relationships with families. Through effective communication, empathy, and collaboration, SDM can transform pediatric care into a more inclusive and patient-centered practice.

8

GUIDANCE FOR PEDIATRIC TRAINEES

Best Practices in Pediatric Healthcare from Internship to Residency

Pediatric internship and residency programs serve as the foundation for healthcare professionals embarking on careers in pediatric medicine.

The best practices of pediatric healthcare, starting from internship through residency training, must include clinical excellence, compassionate care, and professional development, empowering pediatric trainees to become competent and compassionate pediatric healthcare providers.

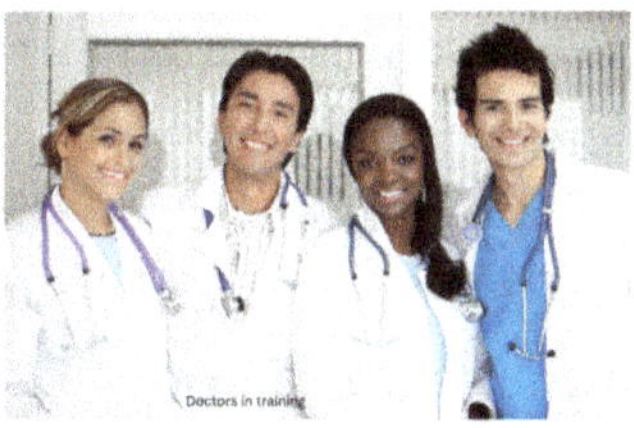

Navigating Pediatric Internship

Guidance for pediatric interns as they transition into clinical practice is very important as new healthcare providers learn how a good and acceptable bedside manner is laid or established and developed with the mastering of basic clinical skills to develop effective communication strategies, which will result in patient trust, compliance, and satisfaction, and provider transparency and professional rapport.

Clinical Excellence in Pediatric Care

Clinical excellence is the cornerstone of pediatric healthcare.

- **Guidance for Pediatric Trainees**:
    - **Goal Setting**: Trainees should identify short-term and long-term goals, from completing specific clinical competencies to presenting research. Clear goals allow for focus and motivation, setting a clear path toward their career aspirations.
    - **Seeking Mentorship**: Mentorship helps trainees develop clinical skills, professional insights, and networking connections. Finding a mentor who aligns with a trainee's interests and values provides valuable guidance, support, and growth opportunities.
    - **Cultivating a Growth Mindset**: Encouraging resilience and a willingness to learn from setbacks is essential in pediatric practice. Trainees benefit from seeing challenges as opportunities for growth, ultimately strengthening their clinical skills and adaptability.

STRATEGIES FOR MANAGING STRESS

3. Strategies for Managing Stress, Preventing Burnout, and Promoting Resilience in Pediatric Practice

- **Time Management and Work-Life Balance**: Maintaining a healthy work-life balance is crucial. Time management skills, such as setting priorities and using digital tools to organize tasks, help avoid overwhelming workloads.
- **Self-Care and Mindfulness**: Practicing self-care is essential to maintaining mental and physical health. Regular exercise, mindfulness practices, and relaxation techniques help reduce stress levels and increase resilience.
- **Building Support Networks**: Engaging with peers, family, and mentors provides emotional support, especially during challenging times. Support networks help prevent feelings of isolation, which can contribute to burnout.

- **Boundary Setting**: Establishing healthy boundaries between work and personal life prevents over-commitment, which can lead to exhaustion. Practitioners should prioritize time off, limit after-hours communication, and advocate for reasonable caseloads.
- **Recognizing Burnout Symptoms**: Symptoms of burnout, such as fatigue, detachment, and a reduced sense of accomplishment, should not be ignored. Encouraging open discussions about mental health and making use of counseling services can help address burnout early.

RESOURCES AND SUPPORT SYSTEMS FOR PEDIATRIC TRAINEE

4. Resources and Support Systems for Pediatric Trainees

- **Educational Resources**: Pediatric trainees have access to a wealth of resources, from online medical libraries (e.g., UpToDate, PubMed) to specialty-focused platforms (e.g., Pediatric Care Online by the AAP). These resources provide ongoing learning and evidence-based practice guidelines.
- **Wellness Programs**: Many medical institutions offer wellness programs, which might include mental health services, fitness resources, and stress management workshops tailored to the needs of healthcare providers.
- **Residency and Fellowship Support**: Structured residency and fellowship programs often include professional development courses, workshops on work-life balance, and access to mental health services, helping trainees navigate the stresses of early practice.
- **Peer Support Groups**: Informal or formal peer support groups allow trainees to share experiences, discuss challenges, and gain insights from colleagues facing similar situations.

These groups promote camaraderie and resilience within the pediatric field.

By fostering healthy habits, preventing disease, and addressing developmental concerns, pediatric providers support children's health, well-being, and development. Additionally, lifelong learning, mentorship, resilience-building, and stress management enable pediatric providers and trainees to thrive professionally and deliver high-quality care for their young patients.

1. Strategies for Providing High-Quality, Evidence-Based Care in Pediatrics

• **Accurate Diagnosis and Appropriate Treatment**:

o **Evidence-Based Practice**: Utilizing up-to-date, evidence-based guidelines and research when diagnosing and treating pediatric patients helps ensure that care aligns with the latest findings in child health.

o **Age-Appropriate Diagnostics**: Pediatric patients vary greatly in physiology and development; diagnostic tools, tests, and treatment plans should be tailored to a child's specific age, developmental stage, and medical history.

o **Family-Centered Care**: Integrating family insights and preferences into care planning recognizes the family's role in a child's health, helping build treatment plans that consider lifestyle and family dynamics for better adherence and outcomes.

• **Effective Care Coordination**:

o **Collaborative Approach**: Coordinating care among pediatric specialists, primary care providers, and allied health professionals (e.g., nutritionists and occupational therapists) creates a holistic approach that addresses the broad range of pediatric health needs.

o **Clear Communication Channels**: Establishing efficient communication between caregivers and healthcare providers ensures continuity of care and helps prevent gaps or duplications in treatment.

o **Use of Health Technology**: Electronic health records (EHRs), patient portals, and telehealth can streamline care coordination, allowing providers to track and share information seamlessly while offering families more convenient access to care.

• **Principles of Clinical Excellence in Pediatric Medicine**:

o **Commitment to Best Practices**: Providers should prioritize clinical excellence by engaging in continuous learning, participating in peer reviews, and adopting standardized clinical guidelines.

o **Patient Safety**: Pediatric care must emphasize minimizing risk, managing potential complications, and adhering to protocols designed to ensure safety in all healthcare interactions.

o **Empathy and Compassion**: A compassionate approach builds trust, reduces anxiety in young patients, and positively influences their overall healthcare experience.

2. Importance of Building Strong Patient-Provider Relationships

• **Trust and Open Communication**: Children and their families often feel more comfortable and open with providers who take the time to listen, address concerns, and explain medical information in an accessible way.

• **Long-Term Health Outcomes**: Positive relationships encourage regular check-ups, follow-through on treatment plans, and early intervention when new symptoms arise, all of which improve long-term health outcomes.

• **Patient and Family Engagement**: Involving patients and families in care planning and decision-making leads to more personalized care and greater adherence to prescribed treatments, as patients feel their values and preferences are acknowledged.

• **Building a Sense of Security**: For young patients, especially, establishing trust in their healthcare provider helps reduce fears related to clinical settings, supporting a healthier outlook on medical care over their lifetime.

3. Embracing Diversity and Cultural Competence in Pediatric Care

• **Importance of Cultural Competence**:

- **Providing Inclusive Care**: Cultural competence ensures that care is respectful of and responsive to the beliefs, practices, and values of diverse patient populations. It is essential to create a welcoming environment where all patients feel understood and respected.
- **Reducing Health Disparities**: Culturally competent care can help address and reduce health disparities by understanding and adapting to the specific needs of various cultural groups, which in turn improves health equity.
- **Supporting Better Health Outcomes**: When patients and families feel that their cultural needs and perspectives are honored, they are more likely to engage with healthcare services and follow treatment recommendations.

• **Key Components of Cultural Competence**:

◦ **Cultural Humility**: Providers should approach each patient interaction with openness, self-awareness, and a willingness to learn from the patient's perspective, rather than assuming knowledge based on generalizations.

◦ **Sensitivity to Cultural Norms**: Understanding cultural

differences in concepts of illness, family roles, and decision-making processes helps providers build rapport and avoid unintentional misunderstandings.

◦ **Effective Cross-Cultural Communication**: Using clear, respectful language, acknowledging differences, and addressing any language barriers through interpreter services when necessary are crucial for building understanding and trust.

4. Strategies for Promoting Diversity, Equity, and Inclusion in Pediatric Training Programs

• **Recruitment of Diverse Trainees**: Proactively recruiting residents and fellows from a variety of backgrounds brings diverse perspectives and experiences to the pediatric field, helping address health inequities and enhance culturally competent care.

• **Incorporating DEI into Curricula**: Pediatric training programs should integrate diversity, equity, and inclusion (DEI) education into their curricula, covering topics such as implicit bias, health disparities, and strategies for inclusive care.

• **Cultural Competency Training**: Providing workshops and continuous learning opportunities on cultural competence and humility helps trainees recognize and address personal biases and understand the importance of inclusive, patient-centered care.

• **Mentorship Programs for Underrepresented Trainees**: Establishing mentorship programs that support underrepresented medical trainees can help them navigate challenges in the medical profession, offering role models and guidance that promote retention and success.

Encouraging Community Engagement: Exposing trainees to community outreach initiatives allows them to interact with diverse populations in non-clinical settings, fostering a deeper understanding of the social determinants of health and the unique needs of underserved communities.

Prioritizing these strategies in pediatric care promotes high standards of clinical excellence, supports strong patient-provider relationships, and ensures that all children receive compassionate, equitable care. By championing diversity, equity, and inclusion, pediatric providers and training programs can work together to create a healthcare environment where every child feels safe, understood, and empowered to lead a healthy life.

Preventive Care and Health Promotion

Preventive care and health promotion are essential components of pediatric practice.

1. Strategies for Promoting Healthy Behaviors in Pediatric Patients

- **Parental Education and Involvement**: Parents and caregivers are essential partners in promoting children's healthy habits. Healthcare providers can educate parents on age-appropriate nutrition, exercise, sleep routines, and screen time management.
- **Modeling and Reinforcement**: Encouraging parents to model healthy behaviors, such as physical activity, healthy eating, and stress management, helps children see these habits as part of their daily lives. Providers can offer positive reinforcement for families practicing healthy behaviors.
- **Setting Achievable Goals**: Working with children and families to set small, achievable goals helps build momentum. Goals can include specific activities like "20 minutes of outdoor play each day" or "five servings of fruits and vegetables daily."
- **School and Community Engagement**: Partnering with

schools and community organizations can amplify health promotion efforts. Programs that provide healthy meals, physical activity sessions, and mental health support reach children in broader community contexts, promoting healthy behaviors on a larger scale.

• **Technology and Tools**: Using apps, educational videos, and interactive platforms can engage children and their families in learning about health. Providers might recommend tools that track activity, reinforce learning about healthy food choices, or promote mindfulness.

2. Preventing Disease in Pediatric Patients

• **Vaccination and Immunization**: Timely vaccinations are foundational in preventing serious infectious diseases. Providers should ensure children stay up-to-date on recommended vaccines, offering education on vaccine safety and addressing parental concerns.

• **Nutritional Guidance**: Good nutrition supports a child's immune system, growth, and development. Providers should emphasize a balanced diet with adequate vitamins and minerals, limit processed foods, and encourage hydration.

• **Oral Health**: Preventing dental diseases through regular brushing, flossing, and routine dental check-ups is critical. Educating parents on limiting sugary foods and drinks and reinforcing the importance of dental hygiene from an early age helps maintain oral health.

• **Physical Activity and Sedentary Behavior**: Encouraging physical activity supports children's cardiovascular health, mental well-being, and physical fitness. For young children, play-based activities promote movement, while older children can engage in sports, dance, and other structured activities.

• **Safe Environments**: Disease prevention also involves promoting safety measures such as car seat use, helmet-wearing for bicycles, and supervision during play. Educating families on injury prevention is an integral part of preventive care.

3. Addressing Developmental and Behavioral Concerns in Pediatric Patients

- **Developmental Screenings**: Regular screenings help identify developmental delays in areas like language, motor skills, socialization, and cognition. These screenings allow for early referrals to specialists if needed, which can significantly improve outcomes.
- **Behavioral Health Support**: Addressing behavioral issues early can prevent escalation and improve coping skills. For concerns like ADHD, anxiety, or depression, early counseling, behavioral therapy, or family education can support the child's well-being.
- **Parental Support and Resources**: Providing resources for parents, such as parenting workshops or materials on managing challenging behaviors, can empower families to handle developmental or behavioral issues proactively.
- **Integrated Care Teams**: Multidisciplinary teams that include psychologists, therapists, and social workers alongside pediatricians are effective in managing developmental and behavioral issues holistically, ensuring that children and their families have comprehensive support.

4. Importance of Early Intervention, Screening, and Anticipatory Guidance in Pediatric Healthcare

- **Early Intervention**:
    - Early intervention for developmental or behavioral issues can lead to better long-term outcomes. For instance, children diagnosed with speech or motor delays benefit from therapy during critical developmental periods.
    - Intervening early in cases of obesity, asthma, or behavioral concerns helps mitigate the likelihood of these issues

continuing into adulthood, reducing the risk of chronic disease and promoting a better quality of life.

- **Screening**:
  - **Routine Screenings**: Screenings at well-child visits help identify developmental, physical, and behavioral issues that may require further attention. These screenings include vision, hearing, developmental milestones, and behavioral health assessments.
  - **Targeted Screenings**: In addition to general developmental screenings, targeted screenings for conditions like autism, depression, and anxiety help identify issues that may not be immediately visible. This approach allows for timely referrals to specialists if needed.
- **Anticipatory Guidance**:

- **Guiding Parents**: Anticipatory guidance provides parents with information on what to expect in their child's development and how to handle upcoming challenges. For instance, advising parents on toilet training, dealing with picky eating, or managing screen time helps them prepare for their child's developmental stages.
- **Encouraging Healthy Lifestyles**: Anticipatory guidance also includes promoting habits like safe sleep, regular physical activity, and balanced nutrition. By educating families early, providers can help establish a foundation for lifelong health.
- **Building Resilience**: Providers can help families build resilience by encouraging strong social connections, routines, and coping strategies, which support mental health and well-being in the face of future stressors.

The strategies above illustrate the comprehensive approach needed to support pediatric patients, from early screenings to guidance on healthy behaviors. By providing education, support, and early interventions, healthcare providers play a key role in fostering the health, development, and well-being of children.

1. Strategies for Promoting Healthy Behaviors, Preventing Disease, and Addressing Developmental and Behavioral Concerns in Pediatrics

- **Promoting Healthy Behaviors**:
  - **Nutrition and Exercise Education**: Providers can guide families in understanding the importance of balanced nutrition, regular physical activity, and adequate sleep for children. Setting age-appropriate health goals, such as reducing sugary drinks or incorporating daily play, reinforces these behaviors.
  - **Positive Role Modeling**: Encouraging parents and caregivers to model healthy behaviors, such as eating nutritious foods and engaging in physical activities, helps children see these habits as a normal part of life.
  - **Parental Involvement and Family-Based Interventions**: Healthy behaviors are more likely to be adopted when the whole family participates. Teaching families simple ways to prepare healthy meals or create exercise routines can strengthen engagement.
  - **School and Community Programs**: Partnering with local schools or community organizations to organize health education events, physical activities, or wellness challenges that reach children in broader contexts.
- **Preventing Disease**:
  - **Vaccination Programs**: Regular immunizations are essential for preventing infectious diseases. Providers can support parents by educating them on vaccine safety and effectiveness and addressing common concerns.

- ◦ **Routine Health Screenings**: Annual check-ups with screenings for vision, hearing, and overall development help catch issues early. Specific screenings, like those for anemia, lead exposure, or high cholesterol (for at-risk populations), play a role in preventive care.
- **Injury and Environmental Safety**: Educating families about safety practices—such as the proper use of car seats, helmets, and environmental hazard awareness (e.g., smoke detectors, lead exposure)—helps reduce preventable injuries and illnesses.

- **Addressing Developmental and Behavioral Concerns**:
  - **Early Developmental Screenings**: Developmental assessments can identify delays early on, allowing for timely referrals to specialists in speech therapy, occupational therapy, or behavioral therapy as needed.
  - **Behavioral Health Screening**: Screening for behavioral health concerns like anxiety, depression, and ADHD is crucial. Connecting families with counseling, family therapy, or social work resources provides targeted support.
  - **Parental Resources and Education**: Providing educational materials on child development and behavioral management techniques empowers parents to support their children effectively.
- **Importance of Early Intervention, Screening, and Anticipatory Guidance**:
  - **Early Intervention**: Early intervention in developmental, physical, or behavioral concerns can lead to more favorable outcomes. Children who receive early support for developmental delays, for instance, often have improved long-term social and academic outcomes.
  - **Anticipatory Guidance**: Preparing families for developmental stages, safety precautions, and preventive health

measures (e.g., limiting screen time and managing sleep hygiene) fosters proactive, informed parenting.

2. Continuing Medical Education and Participation in Professional Organizations

- **Importance of Lifelong Learning**: Pediatric medicine evolves constantly, so continuing medical education (CME) ensures providers remain current with best practices and innovations in the field. Through workshops, seminars, and online courses, practitioners can update their knowledge of new treatments, diagnostic tools, and evidence-based care strategies.
- **Benefits of Professional Organizations**: Membership in organizations like the American Academy of Pediatrics (AAP) offers access to research, professional development courses, conferences, and a supportive network of peers. Staying active in such organizations fosters community involvement and provides access to valuable clinical resources.

9

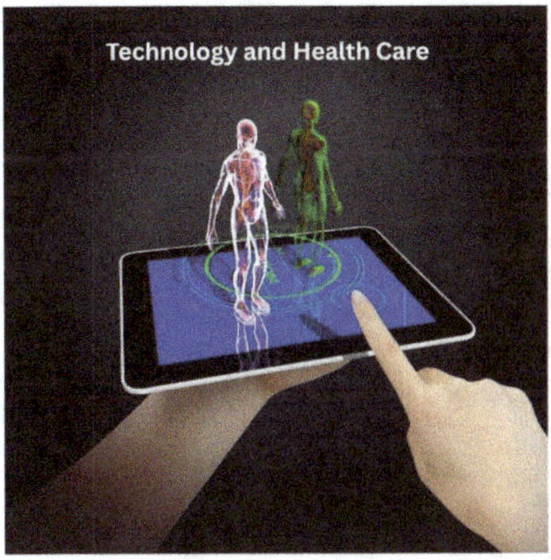

INNOVATING CARE: IMPACT OF TECHNOLOGY

Innovating Care: The Impact of Technology on Best Practices in Pediatric Healthcare

Technology has revolutionized the landscape of pediatric healthcare, offering unprecedented opportunities to improve patient outcomes, enhance efficiency, and advance medical knowledge. Technology is transforming pediatric healthcare by enhancing diagnostic precision, enabling personalized treatment plans, improving patient and family engagement, and advancing research efforts. By harnessing these advancements, pediatric providers can deliver safer, more effective care, leading to better health outcomes and quality of life for children. Here's a breakdown of how technology is reshaping best practices in pediatric healthcare:

1. Enhancing Diagnosis and Treatment in Pediatrics

- **Precision Diagnostics**:
  - **Imaging Technologies**: Advances in imaging, such as MRI and ultrasound, provide high-resolution insights into pediatric conditions

with greater accuracy and less radiation exposure, which is particularly beneficial for children. These technologies help diagnose everything from congenital heart defects to neurological disorders with minimal discomfort for young patients.

  - **Genomic and Genetic Testing**: Genetic testing can reveal predispositions to diseases, allowing for earlier interventions and more accurate diagnoses of rare genetic disorders in children. These technologies enable personalized treatment plans, tailored to a child's unique genetic profile, which increases treatment efficacy.
  - **Artificial Intelligence (AI) and Machine Learning (ML)**: AI is being integrated into diagnostics, especially in interpreting imaging, pathology, and lab results. In pediatrics, AI assists in identifying patterns that indicate specific health conditions, supporting early and accurate diagnoses. AI tools are also used in predicting the course of diseases and optimizing treatment pathways for pediatric patients.

- **Telemedicine and Remote Patient Monitoring**:
  - **Telehealth Platforms**: Telemedicine has expanded access to pediatric care, particularly in rural or underserved areas, allowing children to receive specialized consultations without extensive travel. This is especially useful for routine follow-ups, behavioral health sessions, and management of chronic conditions.

- **Wearable Devices**: Wearable technology, such as pediatric heart monitors, glucose sensors, or smart thermometers, allows for continuous monitoring and real-time alerts. This data helps providers track a child's health trends over time and make timely adjustments to treatment plans as needed, empowering families to be more actively involved in managing their child's health.

- **Robotics and Minimally Invasive Procedures**:
  - Robotics is enabling precision in minimally invasive surgeries, reducing recovery times and lowering the risk of complications in pediatric patients. For example, robot-assisted laparoscopic procedures help decrease pain and speed recovery, making surgery safer and less daunting for children and their families.

IMPROVING PATIENT HEALTH

2. Improving Patient Engagement and Family-Centered Care

- **Patient Portals and Mobile Apps**:
    - Digital patient portals allow families to access their child's medical records, schedule appointments, and communicate with providers. This transparency encourages parents to be more engaged in their child's healthcare, making it easier to track immunizations, receive personalized health tips, and follow treatment plans.
    - Mobile health apps designed for children make health education engaging through interactive tools that teach young patients about their conditions and medications. This can be especially helpful in managing chronic illnesses, like asthma or diabetes, where treatment adherence is essential.

- **Virtual Reality (VR) for Patient Education and Stress Reduction**:
  - VR technology is being used to reduce anxiety in pediatric patients, particularly during medical procedures. By immersing children in calming or entertaining virtual environments, VR can distract from discomfort and ease the stress associated with medical care.
  - VR and augmented reality (AR) tools help educate children and parents about medical procedures, helping demystify complex concepts and creating a better understanding of what to expect, which builds trust and reduces fear.

3. Advancing Pediatric Research and Innovation

- **Big Data and Predictive Analytics**:
  - With electronic health records (EHRs) and other digital data sources, researchers have access to large datasets that reveal patterns in pediatric health, leading to better insights into disease trends and risk factors. For instance, predictive analytics can help identify children at high risk for certain conditions, enabling preventive interventions.
  - Big data also allows researchers to track the effectiveness of treatments across large populations, paving the way for continuous improvement in pediatric care protocols.

- **Clinical Trials and Real-World Evidence**:

    - Digital tools for clinical trial recruitment and data collection have streamlined the research process, making it easier to conduct trials specifically for pediatric populations, which are often underrepresented. By simplifying patient recruitment and remote data collection, researchers can gather insights without placing undue burden on young patients.
    - Real-world evidence tools, which collect data on how treatments perform outside of controlled trials, are providing invaluable information on treatment efficacy and side effects, enabling more personalized and safer pediatric treatments.
- **Artificial Intelligence in Drug Development**:
    - AI accelerates the drug discovery process, analyzing data to identify new therapeutic targets for pediatric diseases. By optimizing this process, AI can shorten the time to market essential medications tailored for children, particularly for rare or complex conditions.

4. Ensuring Safer, More Effective Pediatric Care through Technology

- **EHRs and Care Coordination**: Electronic Health Records (EHRs) play a critical role in consolidating a child's health information, making it easier for providers to access a comprehensive view of each patient's medical history. EHRs enhance care coordination, enabling better communication between primary care providers, specialists, and families.

- **Decision Support Systems**: Clinical decision support systems (CDSS) integrated with EHRs provide real-time guidance to pediatricians, including alerts for drug interactions, dosing adjustments, and personalized treatment suggestions. These systems are particularly valuable in pediatrics, where dosing and treatment protocols vary significantly by age and weight.
- **Remote Access to Specialty Care**: Telemedicine and remote consult platforms make it easier for pediatricians to connect with specialists in real time, ensuring that children receive timely and expert care for complex or rare conditions, regardless of geographic location.

5. Future of Technology in Pediatric Healthcare: Building a Healthier Generation

- **Predictive and Preventive Healthcare**: With tools like genetic testing, AI-driven analytics, and wearable health devices, the future of pediatric care is shifting toward predicting potential health issues before they become critical. This proactive approach could lead to the early detection and prevention of chronic conditions such as diabetes, obesity, or asthma.
- **Personalized Pediatric Medicine**: As technology evolves, pediatric care will continue moving toward tailored treatments based on genetic, environmental, and lifestyle factors unique to each child. This will enable a more customized approach, reducing trial-and-error in treatments and minimizing side effects.

- **Equity in Access to Pediatric Technology**: By expanding telehealth infrastructure and creating low-cost health monitoring solutions, technology can play a vital role in reducing healthcare disparities. Ensuring that all children, regardless of socioeconomic background, have access to technology-based care will help address health inequities in pediatric populations.

Through these innovations, technology is reshaping the landscape of pediatric healthcare. It enables healthcare providers to deliver more effective, timely, and patient-centered care, and it fosters engagement among young patients and their families. By continuing to embrace technological advancements, pediatric healthcare providers are building a future where children have access to cutting-edge treatments and tools that support healthier, brighter futures.

DIGITAL HEALTH

Digital Health Revolution

The digital health revolution has introduced a wealth of innovative technologies into healthcare, each with unique implications for pediatric care. From electronic health records (EHRs) and telemedicine to wearable devices and mobile health apps, these tools are transforming the landscape of pediatric medicine. They promise to improve access, efficiency, and quality of care for children and adolescents, addressing some of the longstanding challenges in pediatric healthcare delivery.

Electronic Health Records (EHRs)

EHRs have become foundational in healthcare, enabling providers to easily access a patient's medical history, lab results, immunization records, and other critical health information. In pediatrics, where continuity of care from infancy through adolescence is vital, EHRs improve care coordination by allowing different providers to share information seamlessly. This is especially important for children with chronic illnesses who require regular follow-ups and multiple specialists. EHRs can also help ensure that children receive age-appropriate screenings and vaccinations, reducing the risk of preventable diseases.

Telemedicine

Telemedicine has revolutionized access to pediatric care, especially for families in rural or underserved areas. With telemedicine, families can consult pediatric specialists without the need to travel long distances, which is particularly beneficial in pediatric specialties like neurology, cardiology, and behavioral health. During the COVID-19 pandemic, telemedicine proved essential for maintaining continuity of care, and it continues to be a critical tool for managing chronic conditions and mental health concerns in children. Telemedicine can also help in acute care situations, providing parents with peace of mind and reducing unnecessary visits to the emergency room.

Wearable Devices

Wearable devices, such as fitness trackers, heart rate monitors, and sleep trackers, are becoming more popular in pediatric care. For children with conditions like diabetes, asthma, or heart problems, wearable devices offer real-time monitoring, which can lead to early detection of potential issues and better management of chronic conditions. In pediatrics, where patient compliance and parental involvement are essential, these devices can provide valuable data that parents and healthcare providers can use to make more informed care decisions. Wearable devices also encourage physical activity and healthy habits, addressing issues like childhood obesity, which is a growing concern worldwide.

Mobile Health Apps

Mobile health (mHealth) apps provide a range of functions, from tracking developmental milestones to managing chronic conditions. Pediatric-specific apps help parents monitor their child's growth and development, schedule vaccinations, and access medical advice. For adolescents, there are apps to support mental health, promote self-care, and offer guidance on topics like nutrition and exercise. These apps can be a valuable educational resource for both parents and young patients, fostering better understanding and management of health. For providers, mHealth apps offer a direct communication channel with patients and families, helping them stay engaged in care between visits.

Big Data and Predictive Analytics

As pediatric care adopts digital health solutions, the vast amount of data generated can be harnessed for predictive analytics. By analyzing EHR data and real-time information from wearable devices, predictive analytics can identify children at risk of developing certain conditions and enable early intervention. This is especially valuable in preventive pediatric care, where early action can significantly improve outcomes. Analytics can also help with resource allocation, identifying trends in patient populations, and helping healthcare systems prepare for seasonal illnesses or outbreaks.

Implications for Access, Efficiency, and Quality of Care

The digital health revolution has the potential to improve access by overcoming geographic and socioeconomic barriers. Telemedicine, for example, ensures that children in rural or underserved areas have access to specialized care, while mobile health apps bring healthcare resources into the hands of families regardless of location. Digital tools also promote efficiency by streamlining workflows and enabling data sharing between providers, reducing duplicative tests and enhancing care coordination. In terms of quality, digital health technologies facilitate personalized care and proactive management of health conditions, resulting in better patient outcomes.

Challenges and Considerations

Despite the many benefits, digital health in pediatric care is not without challenges. Privacy concerns are particularly important, as children's data is highly sensitive, and providers must comply with stringent regulations. Additionally, technology access disparities still exist, and there is a need to ensure that all families have access to digital health solutions. Training providers and educating families on the appropriate use of digital health tools are also essential to maximize their potential.

Conclusion

The digital health revolution offers an exciting future for pediatric healthcare, with tools that can reshape how we provide care to children and support their lifelong health. By leveraging these technologies, pediatric healthcare providers can deliver more accessible, efficient, and higher-quality care, ultimately improving health outcomes for children and supporting healthier futures.

PRECISION MEDICINE

Precision Medicine in Pediatric Healthcare

Precision medicine is transforming healthcare by allowing treatments to be customized to the unique characteristics of each patient. In pediatrics, this approach holds particular promise, as children's genetic makeup, biomarkers, and environmental factors can all influence how they respond to treatments. With technological advancements like genomic sequencing and bioinformatics, healthcare providers are now equipped to implement precision medicine strategies that are especially effective for children with complex or rare conditions. These targeted therapies can offer better efficacy and fewer side effects than traditional approaches, significantly improving outcomes for young patients.

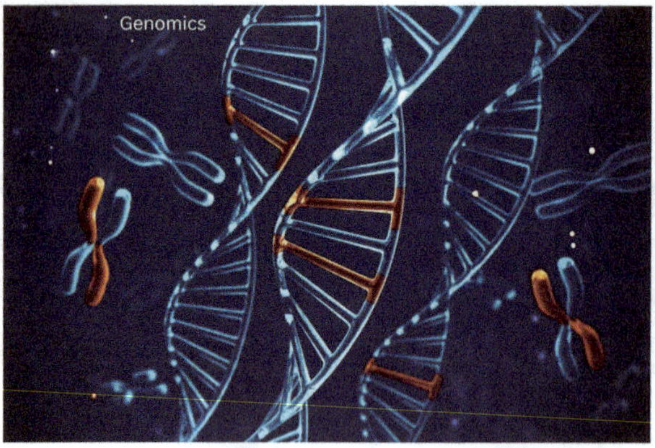

Precision medicine tailors medical care based on an individual's unique genetic profile, lifestyle, and environment. For children, this approach allows for early intervention in genetically predisposed conditions, potentially preventing the onset of diseases later in life. Genomic sequencing—decoding a patient's entire genetic blueprint—is particularly valuable in pediatrics, as it can reveal mutations or genetic markers linked to specific conditions. For example, in oncology, genomic sequencing helps identify the molecular characteristics of tumors, allowing clinicians to select targeted therapies that specifically attack cancer cells while sparing healthy tissue. This personalized approach can also improve the management of other complex pediatric conditions, such as cystic fibrosis, congenital heart defects, and rare genetic disorders, leading to more effective and individualized treatments.

Bioinformatics, which involves analyzing complex biological data, plays a crucial role in precision medicine. By using bioinformatics tools to interpret genetic data, researchers and clinicians can identify potential risk factors, understand disease mechanisms, and develop targeted therapies tailored to a child's unique profile. For instance, bioinformatics has enabled the identification of biomarkers that indicate disease progression or response to treatment, helping clinicians adjust therapies as needed and improving outcomes. These advancements allow for a more proactive and preventive approach to pediatric care, ultimately leading to healthier futures for children.

AI INTEGRATION, DATA PRIVACY, SECURITY, AND BIAS

Artificial Intelligence (AI) and Machine Learning (ML) in Pediatric Care

AI and machine learning are also revolutionizing pediatric healthcare by transforming clinical decision-making, diagnostics, and treatment planning. AI-powered algorithms can process vast amounts of data—such as genetic information, imaging results, and EHR data—more quickly and accurately than human clinicians. By identifying patterns and predicting outcomes, AI can support healthcare providers in making evidence-based decisions, improving the accuracy and efficiency of pediatric care.

In diagnostics, AI algorithms can analyze medical images to detect early signs of diseases, such as pediatric cancers, with high accuracy. For example, AI tools can analyze MRI scans and detect subtle abnormalities that may be missed by the human eye, leading to earlier diagnosis and treatment. AI is also being used to interpret genetic data, aiding in the diagnosis of rare genetic disorders that might otherwise go undetected. In pediatrics, where early intervention is often crucial, AI-driven diagnostics can lead to timely treatment and better outcomes.

AI is also enhancing treatment planning and decision-making. Machine learning models can predict how individual patients will respond to specific treatments based on their genetic profiles and medical histories. This predictive capability allows clinicians to select therapies with the highest likelihood of success, reducing trial and error in treatment. For instance, AI-driven tools can predict the risk of adverse reactions to medications, which is particularly important in pediatric care, where dosing and side effects must be carefully managed. By personalizing treatment in this way, AI can help minimize side effects and improve the overall quality of life for pediatric patients.

Improved Efficiency and Outcomes in Pediatric Care Delivery

The integration of AI and ML in pediatric care offers multiple benefits, including improved efficiency and outcomes. AI can streamline workflows by automating repetitive tasks, such as data entry and analysis, allowing healthcare providers to focus more on patient care. AI algorithms can also continuously learn from new data, adapting and improving over time. For example, predictive models that assess a child's risk for conditions like asthma or diabetes can be refined with additional patient data, leading to even more accurate predictions and early interventions.

Moreover, AI can help identify trends in pediatric populations, providing valuable insights into public health. For example, by analyzing data from wearable devices and health apps, AI can track activity levels, sleep patterns, and other indicators across large groups of children, identifying risk factors for conditions like childhood obesity or anxiety disorders. This information can guide public health initiatives and inform preventive care strategies that benefit entire communities.

Challenges and Future Directions

While precision medicine and AI offer significant potential, their implementation in pediatric care presents unique challenges. Data privacy is a significant concern, as children's genetic and health information must be securely stored and protected. Additionally, ensuring equitable access to these advanced technologies is essential to avoid disparities in care. Training providers and updating healthcare infrastructure to support these innovations are also necessary for widespread adoption.

Despite these challenges, precision medicine and AI-driven solutions are poised to redefine pediatric healthcare. As these technologies continue to evolve, they promise to deliver more personalized, effective, and efficient care, empowering healthcare providers to better address the diverse needs of children. By harnessing the power of genomic insights and AI analytics, pediatric medicine can advance toward a future where each child receives the most precise and optimal care for their unique needs, leading to improved health outcomes and quality of life.

The integration of artificial intelligence (AI) into pediatric healthcare offers enormous potential but also raises key ethical dilemmas that must be addressed to ensure the responsible and equitable use of these technologies. Ethical concerns around data privacy, algorithm bias, and accountability are central to the conversation, particularly because children are a vulnerable population with unique healthcare needs and considerations. Establishing ethical guidelines and regulatory frameworks is essential to mitigate these risks, promoting safe, effective, and fair AI applications in pediatric practice.

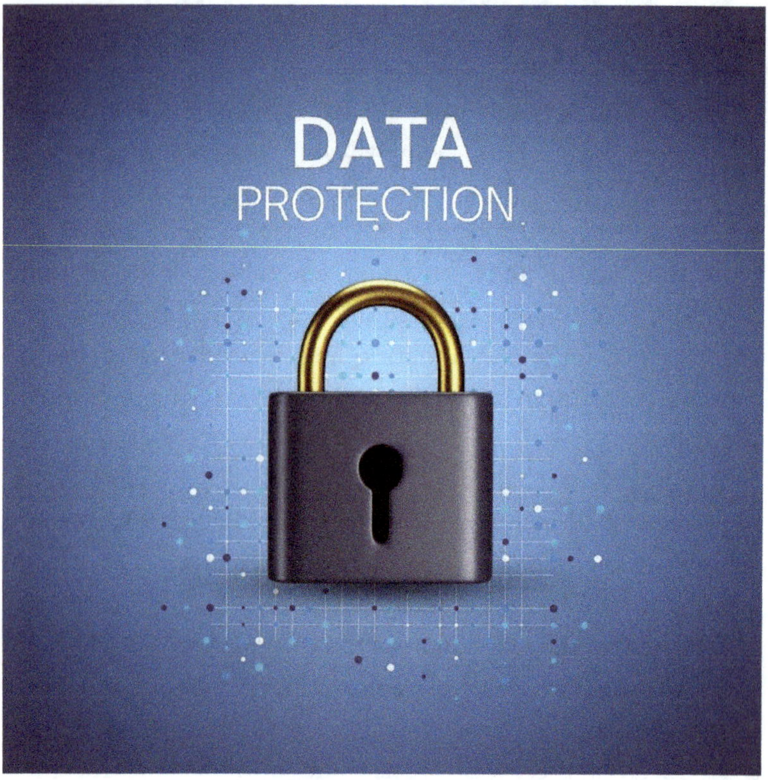

Data Privacy and Security

Data privacy is a critical concern in the application of AI in pediatric healthcare. AI algorithms rely on vast amounts of data, often including sensitive information like genetic profiles, medical histories, and behavioral data, which can be highly identifying, especially in children. Protecting this data is paramount, as breaches could expose children to potential discrimination, future insurance denial, or other forms of harm. Moreover, because children's health data evolves as they grow, there is a unique challenge in managing how this information is stored, accessed, and updated over time.

Ensuring that pediatric data is kept confidential requires stringent security measures and compliance with privacy laws, such as the Health Insurance Portability and Accountability Act (HIPAA) in the U.S. or the General Data Protection Regulation (GDPR) in Europe. However, current regulations often focus on adult data and may not fully address the nuances of pediatric data privacy. Establishing pediatric-specific guidelines for data collection, sharing, and retention could help safeguard children's information, promoting responsible AI use that prioritizes patient confidentiality.

Algorithm Bias and Fairness

Algorithm bias is another ethical challenge in the use of AI for pediatric healthcare. AI systems are trained on historical data, which can inadvertently reflect and perpetuate existing biases in healthcare delivery. For example, if an AI model is trained on a dataset that predominantly includes data from certain demographic groups, it may perform less accurately for children from underrepresented backgrounds. This issue is especially concerning in pediatrics, where accurate diagnoses and treatments are crucial to a child's healthy development.

Addressing algorithm bias requires a multi-pronged approach that includes using diverse datasets, regularly auditing algorithms, and incorporating fairness metrics into AI development. Pediatric AI models should be tested and validated across various demographic groups, including different ages, ethnicities, socioeconomic backgrounds, and geographic locations.

This approach helps ensure that AI tools perform equitably and accurately for all children, regardless of their background. Additionally, ongoing monitoring of AI systems in real-world settings can help detect and correct bias over time, making these tools safer and more effective.

Accountability and Transparency

The question of accountability is central to the ethical use of AI in pediatric care. When an AI system is involved in clinical decision-making, determining who is responsible for any adverse outcomes becomes complex. For instance, if an AI-driven diagnostic tool provides an inaccurate recommendation that leads to harm, should the responsibility

fall on the technology developers, the healthcare provider who used the tool, or the institution that implemented it? Ensuring accountability in such cases is critical to maintaining trust in AI systems and protecting patients.

Transparency is closely linked to accountability. Pediatric AI systems should be designed to be transparent, meaning that healthcare providers and, ideally, patients (or their guardians) should be able to understand how these tools arrive at certain recommendations. This transparency is particularly important for pediatric patients, where parents and caregivers need to be fully informed and involved in decision-making. Developing explainable AI (XAI) models that clearly communicate their reasoning can help clinicians make informed decisions, promote trust, and reduce the risk of relying on "black box" systems that offer limited insights into their functioning.

Importance of Ethical Guidelines and Regulatory Frameworks

To navigate these ethical challenges, establishing robust ethical guidelines and regulatory frameworks for AI in pediatric practice is essential. Clear guidelines can help standardize practices, ensuring that AI tools are developed and used responsibly across different healthcare settings. These frameworks should address the unique aspects of pediatric healthcare, such as parental consent, age-based considerations, and the evolving nature of a child's health information.

Ethical guidelines can also set standards for transparency, privacy, and accountability, creating a foundation for the safe and effective use of AI in pediatrics. For instance, guidelines could outline requirements for bias testing, ensuring that pediatric AI systems undergo rigorous validation across diverse populations. Regulations might also specify transparency standards, mandating that healthcare providers are informed about the limitations and potential risks using AI-driven tools in pediatric care.

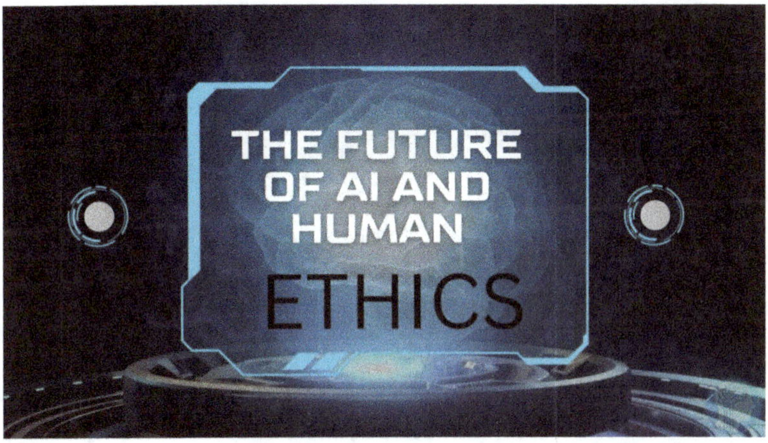

In addition to ethical guidelines, interdisciplinary collaboration among healthcare professionals, technologists, ethicists, and policymakers is vital. By working together, these groups can ensure that AI technologies are designed with pediatric patients' best interests in mind, prioritizing ethical considerations and patient safety throughout the development and deployment processes. Regular review and updates to guidelines are also important to keep pace with technological advancements and evolving ethical standards.

Conclusion

The integration of AI in pediatric healthcare is both promising and complex, raising ethical questions that demand careful consideration and action. Addressing data privacy, algorithm bias, and accountability through clear ethical guidelines and regulatory frameworks is essential to protect young patients and foster the responsible use of AI. With a strong ethical foundation, AI has the potential to transform pediatric healthcare, making it more personalized, accurate, and accessible for all children.

10

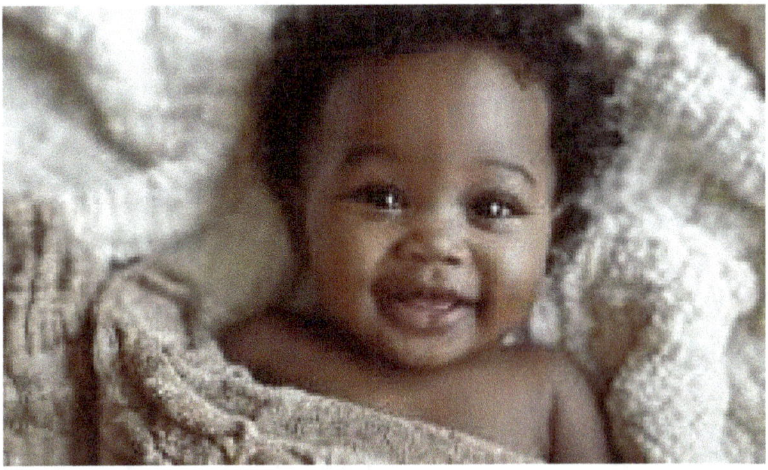

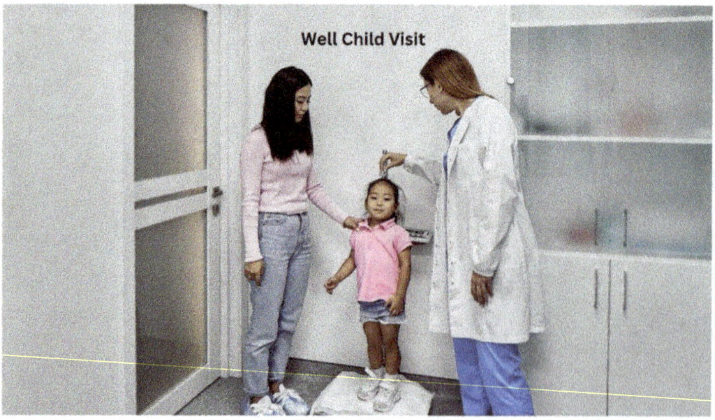
Well Child Visit

WELL CHILD VISIT NEWBORNS

Best Pediatric Practices for Well-Child Visits for Newborns

Introduction- Well-child visits are crucial for monitoring the growth, development, and overall health of newborns. These visits provide an opportunity for pediatricians to offer preventive care, immunizations, and guidance to parents. Chapter 10 outlines the best practices for conducting well-child visits from newborns to 18 years of age, well or sick visits for pediatric patients with single parents, separated or divorced parents, guardianship or State custodial care, suspected neglect or abuse, pediatric patients requiring hospitalization, or behavioral health care, LGBTQIA pediatric patient visits and Adolescent patient visit without a parent, focusing on key aspects such as health assessment, treatment, developmental surveillance, parent education, and preventive care.

1. Initial Health Assessment

A. History Taking

- **Perinatal History**: Document maternal health, pregnancy complications, labor, and delivery details.
- **Family History**: Identify any genetic or familial conditions that may affect the newborn.
- **Social and Environmental History**: Assess the family's living conditions, support systems, and exposure to potential health risks.

B. Physical Examination

Vital Signs: Measure temperature, heart rate, respiratory rate, and oxygen saturation, weight and length

General Appearance: Assess skin color, tone, and overall activity level.

- **Head and Neck**: Check head circumference, fontanelles, eyes, ears, nose, and mouth for abnormalities
- **Cardiorespiratory System**: Auscultate heart and lungs for murmurs, breath sounds, and any abnormalities.
- **Abdomen**: Palpate for organomegaly, and masses, and assess bowel sounds.
- **Genitalia and Anus**: Inspect for normal anatomy and patency.
- **Musculoskeletal System**: Examine the spine, hips, and extremities for deformities or dysplasia.
- **Neurological Assessment**: Evaluate reflexes, muscle tone, and developmental milestones.

2. Developmental Surveillance

A. Growth Monitoring

- **Measurements**: Record weight, length, and head circumference; plot these on standardized growth charts.
- **Trends**: Look for consistent growth patterns; investigate any deviations from expected growth trajectories.

B. Developmental Milestones

- **Motor Skills**: Observe for age-appropriate gross and fine motor development.
- **Social and Emotional Development**: Assess interaction with caregivers, response to stimuli, and bonding behaviors.
- **Cognitive Development**: Monitor alertness, visual and auditory tracking, and early problem-solving skills.
- **3. Parent Education and Guidance**

A. Feeding and Nutrition

- **Breastfeeding Support**: Encourage and support breastfeeding, addressing any challenges and providing resources.
- **Formula Feeding**: Advice on proper formula preparation, feeding techniques, and amounts.
- **Supplementation**: Discuss the need for vitamin D and iron supplementation, as necessary.

B. Sleep and Safety

- **Safe Sleep Practices**: Educate about the importance of placing the baby on their back to sleep, using a firm mattress, and avoiding soft bedding.

- **Car Seat Safety**: Ensure proper car seat installation and usage.
- **Home Safety**: Discuss baby-proofing in the home, safe sleep environments, and the prevention of accidental injuries.

C. Immunizations

- **Schedule**: Review the recommended immunization schedule and administer age-appropriate vaccines.
- **Education**: Provide information about the benefits and possible side effects of vaccines, addressing any parental concerns.

D. Health Promotion

- **Hygiene**: Guide parents on umbilical cord care, bathing practices, and diapering.
- **Oral Health**: Discuss early oral hygiene practices and the importance of avoiding bottle propping.

4. Preventive Care and Screening

A. Newborn Screening Tests

- **Metabolic and Genetic Screening**: Ensure state-mandated newborn screening tests are completed and results are reviewed.
- **Hearing Screening**: Confirm that newborn hearing screening has been performed.

- **Congenital Heart Disease Screening**: Perform pulse oximetry screening to detect critical congenital heart disease.

B. Routine Laboratory Tests

- **Bilirubin Levels**: Monitor for hyperbilirubinemia and assess the need for treatment.
- **Hemoglobin and Hematocrit**: Evaluate for anemia if indicated by risk factors or clinical signs.

5. Follow-Up and Referral

A. Scheduling Next Visit

- **Routine Follow-Ups**: Schedule the next well-child visit according to the recommended timeline (typically at 1 month).
- **Special Concerns**: Arrange earlier follow-up if there are any health concerns or ongoing issues that need closer monitoring.

B. Referrals

- **Specialist Consultation**: Refer to specialists as needed for any identified abnormalities or developmental delays.
- **Community Resources**: Connect families with community resources for additional support, such as lactation consultants, social services, and early intervention programs.

Conclusion

Well-child visits for newborns are a foundational aspect of

pediatric care, ensuring that infants start life with the best possible health and developmental trajectory. By adhering to these best practices, pediatricians can provide comprehensive care that supports the physical, emotional, and developmental well-being of newborns, while also empowering parents with the knowledge and resources they need to care for their child effectively.

WELL CHILD VISIT 2 MONTHS - 5 YEARS

Best Pediatric Practices for Well-Child Visits from 2 Months to 5 Years

Introduction

Well-child visits are critical for monitoring and promoting the healthy development of children from infancy through early childhood. These visits allow pediatricians to assess growth, development, and overall health while providing necessary immunizations and guidance to parents. This section outlines best practices for conducting well-child visits at key age intervals: 2 months, 4 months, 6 months, 9 months, 12 months, 15 months, 18 months, 2 years, 3 years, 4 years, and 5 years.

1. Well-Child Visits at 2 Months

A. Health Assessment

- **History**: Update family history, social environment, and feeding patterns.

- **Physical Examination**: Measure weight, length, and head circumference; assess reflexes, muscle tone, and general health.

B. Developmental Surveillance

- **Milestones:** Look for a social smile, cooing, and head lifting while on the tummy.
- **Growth**: Plot measurements on growth charts and review trends.

C. Parent Education

- **Feeding**: Support breastfeeding or formula feeding; discuss feeding routines.
- **Sleep**: Reinforce safe sleep practices.
- **Immunizations**: Administer the first dose of DTaP, IPV, Hib, PCV20, and rotavirus vaccines.

D. Preventive Care

- **Screening**: Conduct developmental surveillance and discuss any concerns.
- **Safety**: Advice on car seat safety, choking hazards, and home safety.

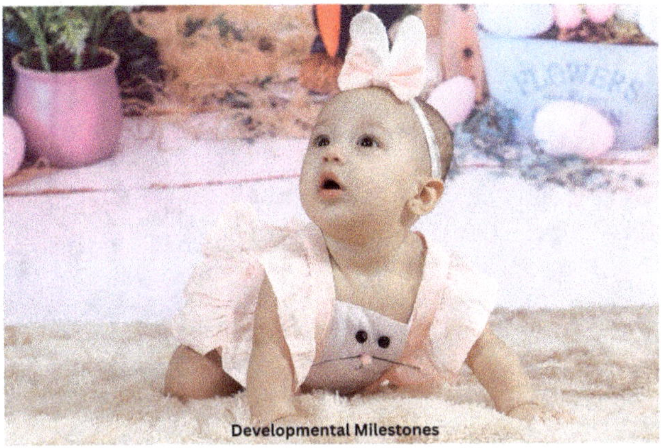
Developmental Milestones

WELL CHILD VISIT 4 MONTHS

2. Well-Child Visits at 4 Months

A. Health Assessment

- **History**: Update feeding patterns, sleep habits, and social history.
- **Physical Examination**: Continue routine measurements and physical exam.

B. Developmental Surveillance

- **Milestones**: Check for head control, reaching for objects, and social interactions.
- **Growth**: Monitor and plot growth metrics.

C. Parent Education

- **Feeding**: Discuss the introduction of solid foods around 6 months.
- **Sleep**: Emphasize routines and safe sleep.

- **Immunizations**: Administer the second dose of DTaP, IPV, Hib, PCV20, and rotavirus vaccines.

D. Preventive Care

- **Screening**: Perform developmental surveillance and address any parental concerns.
- **Safety**: Highlight childproofing and injury prevention.

WELL CHILD VISIT 6 MONTHS

3. Well-Child Visits at 6 Months

A. Health Assessment

- **History**: Review dietary changes, sleep patterns, and family dynamics.
- **Physical Examination**: Conduct a comprehensive physical exam and measurements.

B. Developmental Surveillance

- **Milestones**: Look for sitting with support, babbling, and recognizing familiar faces.
- **Growth**: Continue monitoring growth trends.

C. Parent Education

- **Feeding**: Guide on starting solid foods and allergy prevention.
- **Sleep**: Reinforce consistent sleep routines.

- **Immunizations**: Administer the third dose of DTaP, IPV, Hib, and PCV20 vaccines.

D. Preventive Care

- **Screening**: Developmental surveillance and behavioral observations.
- **Safety**: Advice on safe feeding practices and home safety.

WELL CHILD VISIT 9 MONTHS

4. Well-Child Visits at 9 Months

A. Health Assessment

- **History**: Update on developmental progress, diet, and family interactions.
- **Physical Examination**: Routine measurements and physical assessment.

B. Developmental Surveillance

- **Milestones**: Assess crawling, sitting without support, and responding to names.
- **Growth**: Plot and evaluate growth data.

C. Parent Education

- **Feeding**: Discuss finger foods and variety in the diet.

- **Sleep**: Continue to emphasize sleep safety and routines.
- **Immunizations**: No routine immunizations; catch-up if needed.

D. Preventive Care

- **Screening**: Continue developmental surveillance and discuss any delays.
- **Safety**: Ensure home safety, especially mobility-related hazards.

WELL CHILD VISIT 12 MONTHS

5. Well-Child Visits at 12 Months

A. Health Assessment

- **History**: Update on dietary habits, sleep, and social behaviors.
- **Physical Examination**: Comprehensive physical exam with growth measurements.

B. Developmental Surveillance

- **Milestones**: Look for walking with support, pincer grasp, and simple words.
- **Growth**: Review and plot growth metrics.

C. Parent Education

- **Feeding**: Discuss transitioning to cow's milk and a balanced diet.
- **Sleep**: Maintain safe sleep practices.

- **Immunizations**: Administer MMR, Varicella, Hep A, and final doses of Hib and PCV20

D. Preventive Care

- **Screening**: Conduct lead screening if at risk; developmental surveillance.
- **Safety**: Advice on stair gates, window guards, and continued childproofing.

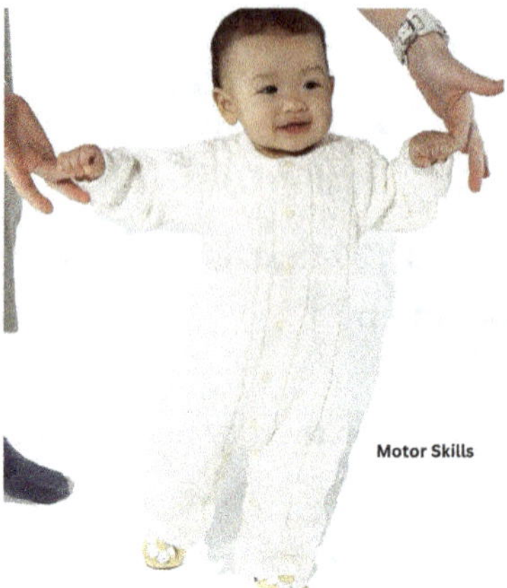

WELL CHILD VISIT 15 MONTHS

6. Well-Child Visits at 15 Months

A. Health Assessment

- **History**: Update on nutrition, sleep, and developmental progress.
- **Physical Examination**: Routine physical exam and growth measurements.

B. Developmental Surveillance

- **Milestones**: Check for walking independently, using a few words, and following simple commands and ask if toddler points at objects he or she wants?
- **Growth**: Continue growth monitoring.

C. Parent Education

- **Feeding**: Discuss a balanced diet and continued introduction of new foods.
- **Sleep**: Emphasize a consistent sleep schedule.
- **Immunizations**: Administer the first dose of DTaP and Hib booster.

D. Preventive Care

- **Screening**: Continue developmental assessments and screenings as needed.
- **Safety**: Discuss poisoning prevention, firearm safety, and outdoor safety.

WELL CHILD VISIT 18 MONTHS

1. **Well-Child Visit at 18 months**
   A. **Health Assessment**

- **History**: Review dietary intake, sleep patterns, and behavioral development.
- **Physical Examination**: Conduct a thorough physical exam and record growth metrics.

B. Developmental Surveillance

- **Milestones**: Assess for running, climbing, increased vocabulary, and pretend play.
- **Growth**: Plot and review growth data.

C. Parent Education

- **Feeding**: Encourage a diverse diet and proper portion sizes.
- **Sleep**: Continue to reinforce regular sleep routines.

- **Immunizations**: Administer Hep A second dose and other catch-up vaccines as needed.

D. Preventive Care

- **Screening**: Developmental screening for autism spectrum disorder (ASD).
- **Safety**: Reinforce childproofing, outdoor safety, and water safety.

WELL CHILD VISIT 2 YEARS

8. Well-Child Visits at 2 Years

A. Health Assessment

- **History**: Update on overall health, development, and family dynamics.
- **Physical Examination**: Routine measurements and physical assessment.

B. Developmental Surveillance

- **Milestones**: Check for running, kicking a ball, two-word sentences, and simple puzzles.
- **Growth**: Monitor and plot growth trends.

C. Parent Education

- **Feeding**: Discuss healthy eating habits and limit sugary foods.
- **Sleep**: Emphasize consistent bedtime routines.

- **Immunizations**: Administer any missed vaccinations.

D. Preventive Care

- **Screening**: Conduct vision screening and developmental surveillance.
- **Safety**: Advice on toilet training, discipline, and household safety.

- **Sleep**: Maintain sleep routines and address sleep issues.
- **Immunizations**: Catch-up vaccines if needed.

WELL CHILD VISIT 3 YEARS

9. Well-Child Visits at 3 Years

A. Health Assessment

- **History**: Review diet, sleep, social, and behavioral development.
- **Physical Examination**: Comprehensive physical exam with growth monitoring

B. Developmental Surveillance

- **Milestones**: Look for climbing, riding a tricycle with a helmet, three-word sentences, and imaginative play.
- **Growth**: Continue to plot and review growth data. Begin blood pressure measurement

C. Parent Education

- **Feeding**: Encourage family meals and balanced nutrition.

- **Sleep**: Maintain sleep routines and address sleep issues.
- **Immunizations**: Catch-up vaccines if needed.

D. Preventive Care

- **Screening**: Vision and hearing screening; developmental assessment.
- **Safety**: Discuss pedestrian safety, water safety, and limit screen time.

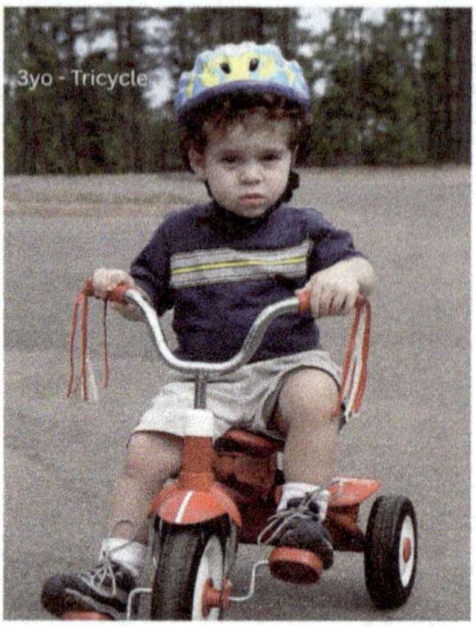

WELL CHILD VISIT 4, 5 YEARS

10. Well-Child Visits at 4 Years

A. Health Assessment

- **History**: Update on nutrition, sleep, and preschool adjustment.
- **Physical Examination**: Routine physical assessment and growth measurements.

B. Developmental Surveillance

- **Milestones**: Assess for hopping, drawing simple shapes, and following multi-step instructions.
- **Growth**: Monitor growth and plot on growth charts.

C. Parent Education

- **Feeding**: Encourage nutritious snacks and regular physical activity.

- **Sleep**: Continue emphasizing good sleep hygiene.
- **Immunizations**: Administer the second dose of MMR and Varicella, and administer the first dose of DTaP and IPV if not previously given.

D. Preventive Care

- **Screening**: Conduct vision and hearing screenings.
- **Safety**: Reinforce safety around strangers, fire safety, and emergency contacts.

11. Well-Child Visits at 5 Years

A. Health Assessment

- **History**: Review overall health, school readiness, and social interactions.
- **Physical Examination**: Comprehensive exam and growth monitoring.

B. Developmental Surveillance

- **Milestones**: Look for skipping, writing some letters, counting, and understanding basic time concepts.
- **Growth**: Continue to monitor and plot growth data.

C. Parent Education

- **Feeding**: Promote healthy eating habits and physical activity.
- **Sleep**: Emphasize regular sleep routines and adequate sleep.

- **Immunizations**: Administer any remaining catch-up vaccines.

D. Preventive Care

- **Screening**: Vision and hearing screening; assess readiness for school.
- **Safety**: Discuss pedestrian safety, booster seat use, and screen time management.

Conclusion

Well-child visits from infancy through early childhood are essential for ensuring optimal growth and development. By following these best practices, pediatricians can provide comprehensive care that supports the physical, cognitive, and emotional well-being of children, while also offering valuable guidance to parents. Regular monitoring, immunizations, and preventive care are key components of these visits, promoting healthy development and early identification of potential issues.

WELL CHILD VISIT
6 YEARS - 8 YEARS

Best Pediatric Practices for Well-Child Visits for Ages 6 to 18

Introduction

Well-child visits from ages 6 to 18 are vital for monitoring the growth, development, and overall health of children and adolescents. These visits provide opportunities to address physical, emotional, and social changes, ensure proper immunizations, and promote healthy behaviors. This section outlines best practices for conducting well-child visits at key developmental stages: 6-8 years, 9-11 years, 12-14 years, and 15-18 years.

1. Well-Child Visits at 6-8 Years

A. Health Assessment

- **History**: Update medical, social, and family history. Inquire about school performance, diet, sleep, and physical activity.

- **Physical Examination**: Conduct comprehensive physical examination including measurement of height, weight, and BMI. Plot growth on standardized growth charts.

B. Developmental Surveillance

- **Milestones**: Assess cognitive skills (reading, math), social interactions (peer relationships), and emotional development (coping skills).

Growth: Monitor growth trends and screen for obesity or growth abnormalities

C. Parent and Child Education

- **Diet and Nutrition**: Discuss a balanced diet, reducing sugary foods, and healthy snacks.
- **Physical Activity**: Encourage regular physical activity and sports participation.
- **Sleep**: Reinforce the importance of adequate sleep (9-12 hours per night).
- **Immunizations**: Ensure vaccinations are up-to-date, including the annual influenza vaccine.

D. Preventive Care

- **Screening**: Conduct vision and hearing screening, and blood pressure measurement, and assess for anemia and lead exposure if at risk.
- **Safety**: Educate about safety measures including bicycle helmet use, car seat/seat belt use, and avoiding exposure to secondhand smoke.

WELL CHILD VISIT
9 YEARS - 11 YEARS

2. Well-Child Visits at 9-11 Years

A. Health Assessment

- **History**: Update on health, school performance, extracurricular activities, and family dynamics. Discuss any concerns about puberty.
- **Physical Examination**: Comprehensive physical exam with growth measurements. Assess for early signs of puberty.

B. Developmental Surveillance

- **Milestones**: Evaluate academic progress, social skills, and emotional well-being.
- **Growth**: Monitor for normal growth patterns and early signs of puberty.

C. Parent and Child Education

- **Diet and Nutrition**: Discuss the importance of a balanced diet and reducing junk food.
- **Physical Activity**: Promote regular exercise and screen time limitations.
- **Sleep**: Emphasize the need for 9-12 hours of sleep per night.
- **Immunizations**: Administer HPV vaccine (starting at age 11), Tdap, and annual influenza vaccine.

D. Preventive Care

- **Screening**: Conduct routine screenings for vision, hearing, and blood pressure, and assess for dyslipidemia if at risk.
- **Safety**: Discuss personal safety, internet safety, and the importance of staying away from drugs and alcohol.

WELL CHILD VISIT
12 YEARS - 14 YEARS

3. Well-Child Visits at 12-14 Years

A. Health Assessment

- **History**: Discuss changes related to puberty, school and social life, behavioral health, and any concerns about substance use.
- **Physical Examination**: Comprehensive exam including assessment of sexual maturation (Tanner staging), growth measurements, and BMI.

B. Developmental Surveillance

- **Milestones**: Assess cognitive development (abstract thinking), emotional health, and peer relationships.
- **Growth**: Monitor growth and development, looking for appropriate progression through puberty.

C. Parent and Child Education

- **Diet and Nutrition**: Encourage a balanced diet rich in fruits, vegetables, and whole grains.
- **Physical Activity**: Recommend at least 60 minutes of physical activity per day.
- **Sleep**: Reinforce the need for 8-10 hours of sleep per night.
- **Immunizations**: Ensure completion of HPV series, Tdap, Meningococcal vaccine, and annual influenza vaccine.

D. Preventive Care

- **Screening**: Screen for depression, substance use, and risk behaviors. Conduct routine vision, hearing, and blood pressure screenings.
- **Safety**: Discuss safe driving, substance abuse prevention, and healthy relationships. Address bullying and cyber safety.

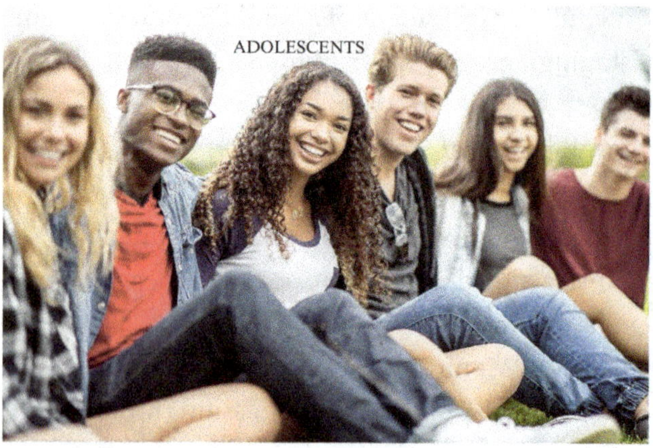

WELL CHILD VISIT
15 YEARS - 18 YEARS

4. Well-Child Visits at 15-18 Years

A. Health Assessment

- **History**: Review academic performance, extracurricular activities, social relationships, behavioral health, and plans for the future.
- **Physical Examination**: Comprehensive physical exam including assessment of sexual maturity, growth measurements, and BMI.

B. Developmental Surveillance

- **Milestones**: Evaluate for academic achievements, career planning, and emotional and social maturity.
- **Growth**: Monitor for completion of growth and development.

C. Parent and Child Education

- **Diet and Nutrition**: Continue to emphasize the importance of a balanced diet and healthy eating habits.
- **Physical Activity**: Encourage regular exercise and involvement in sports or physical activities.
- **Sleep**: Discuss the need for 8-10 hours of sleep per night.
- **Immunizations**: Ensure all adolescent vaccines are up-to-date, including Meningococcal booster and annual influenza vaccine.

D. Preventive Care

- **Screening**: Conduct screenings for behavioral health (depression, anxiety), substance use, sexually transmitted infections (STIs), and routine vision and hearing checks.
- **Safety**: Discuss safe driving practices, substance abuse prevention, safe sexual practices, and healthy relationships. Provide guidance on managing stress and behavioral health.

Conclusion

Well-child visits from ages 6 to 18 are essential for monitoring growth, development, and overall health. These visits allow pediatricians to provide guidance on physical, emotional, and social health, ensure proper immunizations, and promote healthy lifestyle choices. By following these best practices, pediatricians can support the holistic well-being of children and adolescents, preparing them for a healthy adulthood.

11

SICK VISIT – PATIENT OF SINGLE PARENT

Best Practices for Sick Visits for Pediatric Patients of Single Parents

Introduction

Sick visits for pediatric patients of single parents require a compassionate, holistic, and tailored approach to ensure optimal care and support. By focusing on effective communication, personalized treatment plans, proactive follow-up, and holistic support, healthcare providers can address the unique challenges faced by single-parent families. These best practices help ensure that children receive the necessary care and that parents are empowered and supported in their caregiving role.

1. Initial Assessment

A. History Taking

- **Detailed History**: Gather a comprehensive history of the child's current illness, including onset, duration, symptoms, and any treatments attempted. Inquire about previous medical history, allergies, medications, and family medical history.
- **Parental Concerns**: Listen attentively to the parent's

concerns and observations, acknowledging their expertise regarding their child's health.

• **Social and Environmental Context**: Understand the family dynamics, including any stressors that might impact the child's health, such as recent changes in routine, financial issues, or limited access to resources.

B. Physical Examination

• **Thorough Examination**: Conduct a detailed physical examination, focusing on areas relevant to the presenting symptoms. Measure vital signs and assess overall well-being.

• **Developmental and Behavioral Assessment**: Evaluate the child's developmental and behavioral status, as these can influence the presentation and management of illness.

2. Effective Communication

A. Building Rapport

• **Empathy and Understanding**: Show empathy towards the single parent, understanding the unique challenges they may face. Establish a trusting relationship through active listening and validation of their concerns.

• **Clear and Simple Language**: Use clear, non-medical language to explain the diagnosis, treatment plan, and follow-up care. Ensure the parent understands the information provided.

B. Involving the Child

• **Age-Appropriate Communication**: Engage the child in the conversation when appropriate, using age-appropriate language to explain what is happening and what to expect during the visit.

• **Empowerment and Comfort**: Reassure the child, allowing them to express their feelings and fears. Provide comfort and involve them in simple decisions when possible.

3. Tailored Treatment Plans

A. Personalized Care

• **Individualized Treatment**: Develop a treatment plan tailored to the child's specific needs and the family's circumstances. Consider factors such as the parent's work schedule, access to transportation, and financial constraints.

• **Simple and Feasible Interventions**: Recommend treatments that are easy to administer and fit into the family's routine. Provide options for medication administration that accommodate the parent's schedule.

B. Education and Resources

• **Educational Materials**: Provide written instructions and educational materials about the illness, treatment, and when to seek further medical attention. Ensure materials are clear and easy to understand.

• **Access to Resources**: Connect the family with community resources, such as social services, financial assistance programs, and support groups. Provide information on accessing after-hours care or telehealth services if needed.

4. Follow-Up and Continuity of Care

A. Scheduling Follow-Up

• **Flexible Scheduling**: Offer flexible appointment times for follow-up visits to accommodate the parent's work schedule. Consider evening or weekend appointments if possible.

• **Proactive Follow-Up**: Arrange for follow-up calls or visits to monitor the child's progress and address any ongoing concerns. Use telehealth options to reduce the need for in-person visits when appropriate.

B. Coordination of Care

• **Collaborative Approach**: Coordinate care with other healthcare providers, including specialists, therapists, and school nurses, to ensure comprehensive care for the child.

• **Medical Home Model**: Emphasize the importance of a medical home where the child can receive consistent and continuous care. Encourage the single parent to establish a primary care provider relationship for ongoing health needs.

5. Holistic Support

A. Emotional and Social Support

- **Behavioral Health Resources**: Recognize the potential for stress and emotional strain on single parents. Provide referrals to behavioral health resources, counseling services, and parenting support groups.
- **Support Networks**: Encourage the parent to build a support network of family, friends, and community resources. Offer information on local parenting groups and community centers.

B. Empowerment and Advocacy

- **Parent Empowerment**: Empower the single parent by acknowledging their strengths and resilience. Encourage them to advocate for their child's health needs and provide guidance on how to navigate the healthcare system effectively.
- **Educational Workshops**: Offer or recommend workshops and classes on child health, nutrition, and parenting skills to enhance the parent's knowledge and confidence in managing their child's health.

Conclusion

Sick visits for pediatric patients of single parents require a compassionate, holistic, and tailored approach to ensure optimal care and support. By focusing on effective communication, personalized treatment plans, proactive follow-up, and holistic support, healthcare providers can address the unique challenges faced by single-parent families. These best practices help ensure that children receive the necessary care and that parents are empowered and supported in their caregiving role.

SICK VISIT- PATIENT OF SEPARATED/ DIVORCED PARENTS

Best Practices for Sick Visits for Pediatric Patients of Divorced or Separated Parents

Introduction

Sick visits for pediatric patients of divorced or separated parents present unique challenges, including communication between parents, custody arrangements, and emotional stress on the child. This section outlines best practices for conducting sick visits in these situations, emphasizing effective communication, comprehensive assessment, collaborative care planning, and providing holistic support. Providers should remain neutral remaining as advocates for the pediatric patient and avoiding taking sides with either of the parents.

1. Initial Assessment

A. History Taking

- **Detailed Medical History**: Collect a thorough history of the child's current illness, including symptoms, onset, duration, and any previous treatments. Obtain relevant medical history, allergies, and current medications.
- **Parental Input**: Ensure both parents, if involved, have

the opportunity to provide their observations and concerns. Respect custody arrangements and legal considerations regarding medical decisions.

• **Social and Environmental Context**: Understand the child's living situation, including custody arrangements, school environment, and any recent changes or stressors that may impact their health.

B. Physical Examination

• **Comprehensive Examination**: Perform a detailed physical examination, measuring vital signs and assessing the child's overall condition.

• **Developmental and Behavioral Assessment**: Evaluate the child's developmental and behavioral status, considering how emotional stress from family dynamics may affect their health.

2. Effective Communication

A. Building Rapport

• **Empathy and Sensitivity**: Show empathy towards both parents and the child, acknowledging the complexities of their family situation. Establish trust through active listening and validation of their concerns.

• **Clear and Neutral Language**: Use clear, non-biased language when communicating with both parents. Avoid taking sides or making assumptions about family dynamics.

B. Facilitating Communication

• **Involving Both Parents**: Encourage involvement from both parents in the medical discussion and decision-making process, respecting custody agreements. Ensure that both parents receive the same information.

• **Child-Centered Approach**: Engage the child in the conversation where appropriate, using age-appropriate language to explain their condition and treatment.

3. Collaborative Care Planning

A. Developing the Treatment Plan

• **Customized Care**: Tailor the treatment plan to the child's specific needs, taking into account the family's dynamics, custody arrangements, and any logistical challenges.

• **Parental Agreement**: Strive to reach a consensus between both parents regarding the treatment plan. Document agreements and obtain necessary consents as per legal requirements.

B. Education and Resources

• **Clear Instructions**: Provide detailed written instructions about the illness, treatment, and follow-up care. Ensure both parents have copies of all educational materials.

• **Access to Resources**: Offer information on community resources, support groups, and services that can assist with managing the child's health and emotional well-being.

4. Follow-Up and Continuity of Care

A. Scheduling Follow-Up

• **Flexible Scheduling**: Offer flexible appointment times to accommodate the schedules of both parents. Consider evening or weekend appointments if necessary.

• **Proactive Follow-Up**: Arrange follow-up calls or visits to monitor the child's progress and address any ongoing concerns. Use telehealth options to facilitate follow-up when appropriate.

B. Coordination of Care

• **Collaborative Approach**: Coordinate with other healthcare providers, including specialists and school health professionals, to ensure comprehensive and consistent care.

• **Medical Home Model**: Promote the concept of a medical home where the child can receive continuous, coordinated care. Encourage parents to maintain regular contact with the primary care provider.

5. Holistic Support

A. Emotional and Social Support

• **Behavioral Health Resources:** Recognize the potential emotional impact of parental separation on the child. Provide referrals to behavioral health resources, counseling services, and support groups for both the child and parents.

• **Support Networks:** Encourage the establishment of a support network, including extended family, friends, and community resources, to provide additional emotional and practical support.

B. Empowerment and Advocacy

• **Parental Empowerment:** Empower both parents by acknowledging their roles and encouraging collaboration in managing their child's health. Provide guidance on navigating the healthcare system and advocating for their child's needs.

• **Educational Workshops:** Recommend or offer workshops and classes on child health, nutrition, parenting skills, and coping with family changes to enhance parents' knowledge and confidence.

Conclusion

Sick visits for pediatric patients of divorced or separated parents require a thoughtful, collaborative, and compassionate approach. By focusing on effective communication, comprehensive assessment, collaborative care planning, and holistic support, healthcare providers can address the unique challenges faced by these families. These best practices help ensure that children receive the necessary care and support and that parents are empowered and involved in their children's health and well-being.

SICK VISIT- GUARDIANSHIP/ STATE CUSTODIAL CARE

Best Practices for Pediatric Patient Visits in State Custodial or Guardianship Care

Pediatric patients in state custodial or guardianship care often face unique and complex challenges, including emotional trauma, inconsistent medical histories, and multiple caregivers. Providing comprehensive, consistent, and compassionate care for these children requires a specialized approach. This section outlines best practices for conducting medical visits for pediatric patients in state custodial or guardianship care, emphasizing thorough assessment, effective communication, tailored care plans, and holistic support.

1. Initial Assessment

A. History Taking

- **Comprehensive Medical History**: Collect as detailed a medical history as possible, including previous illnesses, surgeries, allergies, medications, and immunization records. Work closely with caseworkers to gather information from previous healthcare providers.

- **Psychosocial History**: Understand the child's current living situation, the reasons for state custody, and any known trauma or behavioral issues. Assess the child's emotional and psychological state.
- **Caregiver Input**: Engage with current caregivers, including foster parents or group home staff, to obtain their observations and concerns about the child's health and well-being.

B. Physical Examination

- **Thorough Examination**: Conduct a detailed physical examination, including measurement of height, weight, and BMI. Assess for any signs of neglect, abuse, or untreated medical conditions.

- **Developmental and Behavioral Assessment**: Evaluate the child's developmental milestones and behavioral health, considering the impact of trauma and instability.

2. Effective Communication
A. Building Rapport

- **Empathy and Trust**: Show empathy and build trust with the child, recognizing the potential for past trauma and mistrust of adults. Use a gentle and reassuring approach.
- **Clear and Compassionate Language**: Communicate clearly and compassionately with

the child and caregivers. Avoid medical jargon and ensure explanations are age-appropriate and understandable.

B. Caregiver Involvement

- **Engage Caregivers**: Involve caregivers in the discussion about the child's health, treatment options, and care plan. Respect their input and provide them with clear instructions and educational materials.
- **Coordination with Caseworkers**: Maintain open communication with caseworkers and other involved professionals to ensure a coordinated approach to the child's care. Share relevant medical information and updates.

3. Tailored Care Plans
A. Personalized Treatment

- **Individualized Care Plans**: Develop individualized care plans that address the specific health needs and circumstances of the child. Consider the child's history, current environment, and potential barriers to care.

- **Feasible Interventions**: Recommend treatments and interventions that are practical and feasible within the child's current living situation. Consider the resources and support available to caregivers.

B. Education and Resources

- **Clear Instructions**: Provide detailed written instructions about the diagnosis, treatment, and follow-up care. Ensure caregivers understand and feel confident in managing the child's health needs.
- **Access to Resources**: Connect caregivers with community resources, support services, and educational materials to assist them in caring for the child. Provide information on accessing after-hours care and emergency services.

4. Follow-Up and Continuity of Care
A. Scheduling Follow-Up

- **Regular Follow-Up**: Schedule regular follow-up visits to monitor the child's progress and address any ongoing health concerns. Ensure appointments are convenient for caregivers and transportation is arranged if needed.
- **Proactive Monitoring**: Implement proactive monitoring through phone calls or telehealth visits to check on the child's well-being between in-person visits.

B. Coordination of Care

- **Multidisciplinary Approach**: Coordinate care with other healthcare providers, behavioral health professionals, educators, and social workers involved in the child's life. Ensure a holistic and integrated approach to care.
- **Medical Home Model**: Advocate for the establishment of a medical home where the child can receive continuous, comprehensive care.

Encourage consistent record-keeping and sharing of medical information.

5. Holistic Support

A. Emotional and Social Support

- **Behavioral Health Resources**: Recognize the high prevalence of behavioral health issues among children in state custody. Provide referrals to behavioral health services, including counseling and therapy, to address trauma and emotional distress.
- **Support Networks**: Encourage the development of a support network for the child, including mentors, supportive adults, and peer groups. Facilitate connections with community organizations and resources.

B. Empowerment and Advocacy

- **Caregiver Empowerment**: Empower caregivers by providing them with the knowledge, resources, and support needed to advocate for the child's health and well-being. Offer training on recognizing and managing common health issues.
- **Child Advocacy**: Advocate for the child's needs within the healthcare system and beyond. Ensure the child's voice is heard and their rights are protected. Work with legal guardians and child welfare agencies to address any systemic issues affecting the child's care.

Conclusion

Caring for pediatric patients in state custodial or guardianship care requires a compassionate, coordinated, and comprehensive approach. By focusing on thorough assessment, effective communication, tailored care plans, and holistic support, healthcare providers can address the unique challenges these children face. Implementing these best practices helps ensure that children in state custody receive the consistent, high-quality care they need to thrive physically, emotionally, and socially.

WELL CHILD VISIT (SUSPECTED ABUSE/NEGLECT)

Best Practices for Well-Child Visits for Pediatric Patients Suspected of Abuse and/or Neglect

Pediatric patients suspected of abuse or neglect require sensitive, comprehensive, and vigilant care during well-child visits. These visits offer critical opportunities to identify and address potential abuse, ensure the child's safety, and provide necessary medical and psychological support. This section outlines best practices for conducting well-child visits for these vulnerable patients, emphasizing thorough assessment, effective communication, multidisciplinary collaboration, and holistic support.

1. Initial Assessment

A. History Taking

- **Detailed Medical History**: Gather a complete medical history, including past illnesses, hospitalizations, surgeries, and any patterns of injury. Carefully document any inconsistencies or unexplained delays in seeking care.
- **Psychosocial History**: Understand the child's living situation, family dynamics, and any known risk factors for abuse

or neglect, such as substance abuse, domestic violence, or behavioral health issues in the family.

• **Behavioral Observations**: Note the child's behavior and interaction with caregivers. Be attentive to signs of fear, anxiety, withdrawal, or overly compliant behavior.

B. Physical Examination

• **Thorough Examination**: Perform a comprehensive physical examination, with particular attention to signs of physical abuse (bruises, burns, fractures) or neglect (poor hygiene, malnutrition, untreated medical conditions).

• **Documentation**: Accurately document all findings with detailed descriptions and, if appropriate and permissible, photographic evidence. Include measurements of injuries and use body charts for precise location mapping.

2. Effective Communication

A. Building Trust

• **Empathy and Sensitivity**: Approach the child with empathy and sensitivity. Use a calm and reassuring manner to help build trust and make the child feel safe.

• **Child-Centered Communication**: Use age-appropriate language and allow the child to express themselves freely. Avoid leading questions and let the child tell their story in their own words.

B. Caregiver Interaction

• **Non-Judgmental Approach**: Maintain a non-judgmental and professional demeanor when interacting with caregivers. Avoid confrontation and focus on gathering information.

• **Private Conversations**: When possible, speak to the child separately from the caregiver to ensure the child can speak freely without fear of repercussion.

1. Multidisciplinary Collaboration

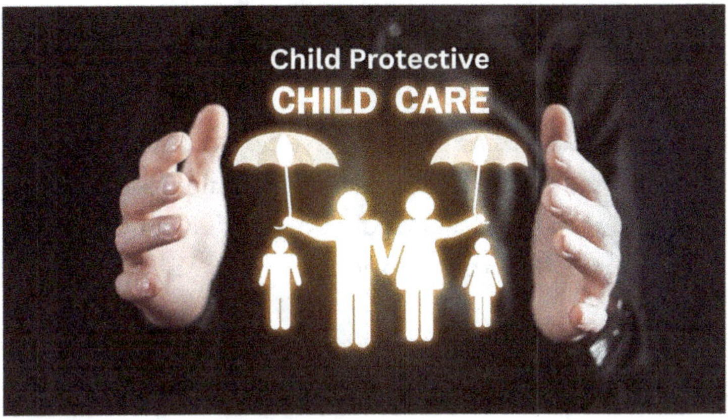

A. Referral and Reporting

- **Mandatory Reporting**: Be aware of mandatory reporting laws and promptly report any suspicions of abuse or neglect to the appropriate child protective services (CPS) or authorities.
- **Referral to Specialists**: Refer the child to relevant specialists, such as pediatric radiologists, child abuse pediatricians, and behavioral health professionals, for further evaluation and support.

B. Coordination with Child Protective Services

- **Collaboration with CPS**: Work closely with CPS and other agencies involved in the child's welfare to ensure a coordinated approach to care and protection.
- **Sharing Information**: Provide detailed medical records and findings to CPS and other involved professionals to support their investigations and interventions.

4. Tailored Care Plans

A. Individualized Care

- **Personalized Approach**: Develop a care plan tailored to the child's specific medical, emotional, and social needs. Consider the child's safety and well-being as the top priority.

- **Follow-Up Care**: Schedule frequent follow-up visits to monitor the child's health, document any new findings, and provide ongoing support.

B. Education and Resources

- **Educational Materials**: Provide caregivers (if safe and appropriate) with educational materials on child health, safety, and positive parenting strategies. Offer resources to help address underlying issues such as substance abuse or behavioral health problems.
- **Support Services**: Connect the family with community resources, such as social services, counseling, and support groups, to provide additional support and assistance.

5. Holistic Support

A. Emotional and Psychological Support

- **Behavioral Health Resources**: Recognize the psychological impact of abuse or neglect. Refer the child to behavioral health professionals for evaluation and therapy to address trauma and emotional distress.

- **Supportive Environment**: Create a supportive and non-threatening environment during visits to help the child feel safe and valued.

B. Empowerment and Advocacy

- **Child Empowerment**: Empower the child by validating their experiences and providing reassurance. Encourage the child to express their feelings and concerns.

- **Advocacy**: Advocate for the child's needs within the healthcare system and beyond. Work with legal representatives and child welfare agencies to ensure the child's rights and best interests are protected.

Conclusion

Well-child visits for pediatric patients suspected of abuse or neglect require a compassionate, vigilant, and multidisciplinary approach. By focusing on thorough assessment, effective communication, collaborative care planning, and holistic support, healthcare providers can play a crucial role in identifying and addressing abuse, ensuring the child's safety, and promoting their overall health and well-being. Implementing these best practices helps create a protective environment where vulnerable children can receive the care and support they need to heal and thrive.

THE PATIENT NEEDING HOSPITALIZATION

Best Practices for Pediatric Patients Needing Hospitalization for Medical Illness

Introduction

Hospitalization can be a stressful experience for pediatric patients and their families. Providing high-quality, compassionate care during hospitalization is crucial for the child's physical and emotional well-being. This section outlines best practices for managing pediatric patients requiring hospitalization for medical illness, emphasizing comprehensive assessment, effective communication, patient-centered care, family involvement, and multidisciplinary collaboration.

1. Admission Process

A. Initial Assessment

- **Comprehensive Medical History**: Obtain a detailed medical history, including current symptoms, past medical history, family history, and any previous hospitalizations. Include information about allergies, medications, and immunization status.
- **Physical Examination**: Perform a thorough physical

examination, documenting vital signs, physical findings, and any immediate medical concerns.

• **Psychosocial History**: Understand the child's living situation, school performance, and any social or emotional stressors. Assess the family's support system and any potential barriers to care.

B. Initial Investigations

- **Diagnostic Tests**: Order appropriate diagnostic tests (e.g., blood tests, imaging) based on the initial assessment to confirm the diagnosis and guide treatment planning.
- **Specialist Consultations**: If needed, arrange for consultations with relevant specialists to provide a comprehensive evaluation and treatment plan.

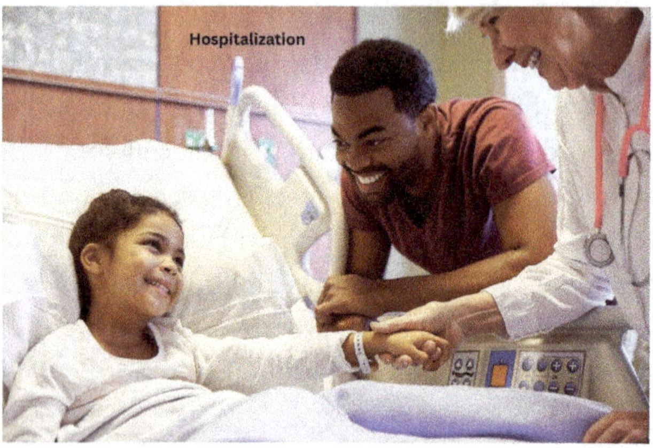

2. Communication and Information Sharing

A. Effective Communication with the Child

- **Age-Appropriate Communication**: Use age-appropriate language to explain the hospitalization process, diagnosis, and treatment plan to the child. Encourage questions and provide reassurance.

- **Emotional Support**: Acknowledge and address the child's fears and anxieties. Offer comfort and support to help them feel safe and understood.

B. Communication with Parents and Caregivers

- **Clear and Consistent Information**: Provide clear, consistent information to parents or caregivers about the child's condition, treatment options, and expected outcomes. Use plain language and avoid medical jargon.
- **Involvement in Decision-Making**: Involve parents or caregivers in the decision-making process, respecting their knowledge and preferences. Ensure they understand and consent to the proposed treatment plan.

3. Patient-Centered Care

A. Individualized Care Plans

• **Personalized Treatment Plans**: Develop individualized care plans based on the child's specific medical needs, preferences, and family circumstances. Consider the child's developmental stage and psychosocial context.

• **Pain Management**: Implement effective pain management strategies, including pharmacologic and non-pharmacologic approaches. Regularly assess and adjust pain management plans as needed.

B. Creating a Child-Friendly Environment

• **Comfort and Familiarity**: Create a child-friendly environment in the hospital, including familiar items from home (e.g., toys and blankets) to provide comfort and a sense of security.

• **Play and Recreation**: Provide opportunities for play and recreational activities to promote normalcy and reduce stress. Utilize child life specialists to support emotional and developmental needs.

4. Family Involvement

A. Supporting Families

• **Family-Centered Care**: Emphasize family-centered care by involving parents and caregivers in all aspects of the child's care. Recognize the family's role as integral to the child's recovery and well-being.

• **Emotional and Practical Support**: Offer emotional support to families, acknowledging the stress and anxiety of hospitalization. Provide practical support, such as information on accommodations, meals, and financial assistance.

B. Education and Resources

• **Health Education**: Educate families about the child's condition, treatment options, and home care requirements. Provide written materials and resources for further information.

• **Discharge Planning**: Begin discharge planning early, ensuring families are prepared for the transition home. Provide clear instructions for follow-up care, medication administration, and signs of potential complications.

5. Multidisciplinary Collaboration

A. Team-Based Care

• **Collaborative Approach**: Foster a collaborative approach to care involving a multidisciplinary team, including physicians, nurses, specialists, child life specialists, social workers, and therapists.

• **Regular Team Meetings**: Hold regular multidisciplinary team meetings to discuss the child's progress, adjust treatment plans, and address any concerns.

B. Coordination of Care

• **Continuity of Care**: Ensure continuity of care by coordinating with primary care providers, specialists, and community resources. Facilitate smooth transitions between different care settings.

• **Documentation and Communication**: Maintain thorough and accurate documentation of the child's medical history, treatment plans, and progress. Ensure clear communication among all team members and with the family.

6. Holistic Support

A. Behavioral Health and Emotional Well-Being

• **Behavioral Health Services**: Screen for behavioral health issues and provide access to behavioral health services, including counseling and therapy, to support the child's emotional well-being.

• **Supportive Interventions**: Use supportive interventions such as art therapy, music therapy, and relaxation techniques to help manage stress and promote healing.

B. Social and Educational Support

• **Educational Continuity**: Ensure educational continuity by coordinating with the child's school and providing hospital-based educational services if needed. Address any academic concerns that may arise during hospitalization.

• **Social Services**: Connect families with social services to address broader social determinants of health, such as housing, food security, and access to community resources.

Conclusion

Hospitalization for pediatric patients requires a compassionate, comprehensive, and family-centered approach. By focusing on thorough assessment, effective communication, individualized care, family involvement, and multidisciplinary collaboration, healthcare providers can ensure that hospitalized children receive the highest quality of care.

Implementing these best practices helps promote the physical and emotional well-being of pediatric patients and supports their families through the challenges of hospitalization.

PATIENT NEEDING BEHAVIORAL HEALTH CARE

Best Practices for Pediatric Patients Needing Behavioral Health Care: Outpatient vs. Inpatient

Introduction

Behavioral health care for pediatric patients requires a thoughtful and comprehensive approach, tailored to the severity and specific needs of each child. Deciding between outpatient and inpatient care depends on various factors, including the child's symptoms, safety, family dynamics, and access to resources. This section outlines best practices for managing pediatric behavioral health care in both outpatient and inpatient settings, emphasizing thorough assessment, effective communication, individualized treatment plans, and holistic support.

1. Assessment and Triage

A. Comprehensive Evaluation

- **Detailed History**: Gather a thorough history of the child's behavioral health, including onset and duration of symptoms, previous behavioral health diagnoses, treatment history, family history, and any trauma or significant life events.

• **Psychosocial Assessment**: Assess the child's living situation, school performance, peer relationships, and family dynamics. Evaluate stressors and supports in the child's environment.

• **Risk Assessment**: Evaluate the risk of harm to self or others, including suicidal ideation, self-harming behaviors, aggressive behaviors, and any history of substance use.

B. Determining Level of Care

• **Criteria for Outpatient Care**: Suitable for children with mild to moderate symptoms, stable home environments, and the ability to attend regular therapy sessions. Outpatient care is appropriate for ongoing management and less severe cases.

• **Criteria for Inpatient Care**: Necessary for children with severe symptoms, acute crises, high risk of self-harm or harm to others, or those needing intensive monitoring and intervention. Inpatient care provides a safe environment for stabilization.

2. Outpatient Care

A. Treatment Planning

Individualized Treatment Plans: Develop tailored treatment plans based on the child's specific needs, preferences, and family circumstances. Include therapeutic interventions, medication management (if needed), and regular follow-up.

• **Evidence-Based Therapies**: Utilize evidence-based therapies such as cognitive-behavioral therapy (CBT), dialectical behavior therapy (DBT), play therapy, and family therapy. Adjust the approach based on the child's developmental stage.

B. Communication and Family Involvement

• **Family Engagement**: Involve parents or caregivers in the treatment process, providing education on the child's condition and how they can support their child. Family therapy may be beneficial to address dynamics and improve communication.

- **Regular Check-Ins**: Schedule consistent follow-up appointments to monitor progress, adjust treatment plans, and address any emerging issues. Use telehealth options to enhance accessibility.

C. Coordination of Care

- **Multidisciplinary Approach**: Collaborate with school counselors, social workers, primary care providers, and other relevant professionals to ensure a coordinated approach to the child's care.

- **Community Resources**: Connect families with community resources, support groups, and educational workshops to provide additional support and information.

3. Inpatient Care

A. Admission Process

- **Thorough Admission Assessment**: Conduct a comprehensive assessment upon admission, including detailed psychiatric evaluation, physical examination, and laboratory tests as needed.

- **Safety and Stabilization**: Prioritize the child's safety and stabilization. Implement measures to prevent self-harm or harm to others and manage any acute psychiatric symptoms.

B. Treatment During Hospitalization

- **Intensive Therapy**: Provide intensive, daily therapeutic interventions, including individual therapy, group therapy, and family therapy. Utilize evidence-based approaches tailored to the child's needs.

- **Medication Management**: Closely monitor and adjust psychiatric medications as needed. Educate the child and family about medication use, side effects, and adherence.

C. Family Involvement and Education

• **Family Participation**: Encourage active participation of family members in the treatment process. Provide education on the child's diagnosis, treatment plan, and strategies to support recovery.

• **Discharge Planning**: Begin discharge planning early, ensuring a smooth transition from inpatient to outpatient care. Develop a comprehensive aftercare plan that includes follow-up appointments, therapy sessions, and community resources.

4. Transition Between Levels of Care

A. Continuity of Care

• **Seamless Transition**: Ensure a seamless transition between inpatient and outpatient care. Communicate clearly between inpatient and outpatient providers to maintain continuity of care.

• **Post-Discharge Support**: Provide intensive support immediately after discharge, including frequent follow-up appointments and crisis intervention if needed. Address any barriers to accessing outpatient care.

B. Monitoring and Follow-Up

• **Regular Monitoring**: Continuously monitor the child's progress and adjust the treatment plan as needed. Ensure that the child is attending follow-up appointments and engaging in prescribed therapies.

• **Crisis Management**: Develop a crisis management plan for the family, including emergency contact information and steps to take if the child's condition deteriorates.

5. Holistic Support and Long-Term Management

A. Addressing Social Determinants of Health

• **Comprehensive Support**: Address broader social determinants of health that may impact the child's behavioral well-being, such as housing, food security, and access to education and extracurricular activities.

- **Support Networks**: Encourage the development of support networks, including peer support groups, community organizations, and mentoring programs.

B. Promoting Resilience and Coping Skills

- **Building Resilience**: Teach and reinforce resilience and coping skills through therapeutic interventions and everyday interactions. Encourage activities that promote self-esteem and a sense of achievement.
- **Ongoing Education**: Provide ongoing education for the child and family about behavioral health, self-care strategies, and how to manage stress and emotions effectively.

Conclusion

Providing behavioral health care for pediatric patients requires a comprehensive, coordinated, and compassionate approach, tailored to the specific needs and circumstances of each child. By distinguishing between the requirements for outpatient and inpatient care, focusing on thorough assessment, effective communication, individualized treatment plans, and holistic support, healthcare providers can ensure that children receive the necessary care to support their behavioral health and overall well-being. Implementing these best practices promotes a stable and supportive environment for children to thrive both during and after treatment.

LGBTQIA+ PEDIATRIC PATIENT VISIT

Best Practices for a Well-Child Visit for a LGBTQIA+ Pediatric Patient

Best practices by healthcare providers for a well-child visit for a LGBTQIA+ pediatric patient play an essential role in offering sensitive, compassionate care to LGBTQIA+ youth, understanding that these patients may face unique challenges related to their sexual orientation and social acceptance. Here are some key best practices for a successful well-child visit:

1. **Creating a Safe Environment**

   - **Display Welcoming Atmosphere**: Having visible symbols such as posters or pamphlets on LGBTQIA+ health in the clinic can make LGBTQIA youth feel welcome.
   - **Neutral Language**: Train staff and providers to use non-assumptive language that respects gender and sexual orientation diversity. This includes terms like "partner" instead of "boyfriend" or "girlfriend,"

which supports a range of orientations and family structures.

- **Pronoun Sensitivity**: Always ask about the patient's preferred pronouns and respect them.

2. Building Trust through Communication

- **Confidentiality**: Reassure patients that their discussions are confidential within the bounds of healthcare privacy laws. LGBTQIA+ youth, particularly those not "out" to family or friends, may worry about privacy, so it's essential to establish and communicate confidentiality.
- **Open Dialogue**: Encourage open and non-judgmental communication. Show genuine interest and respect, asking questions to understand any challenges they may be facing, including social support, behavioral health, and stress.
- **Listen Actively**: Listen to the patient's concerns without rushing. Being heard and validated by a healthcare provider can positively impact their emotional and behavioral health, especially if they feel misunderstood or marginalized outside the clinic.

3. Understanding and Addressing Health Risks

- **Behavioral Health Screening**: LGBTQIA+ youth may have higher rates of anxiety, depression, and other behavioral health challenges due to discrimination or bullying. Regular behavioral health assessments help identify any issues early on. Offer support and, if needed, referrals to LGBTQIA+ competent behavioral health providers.

- **Sexual Health Education**: Provide age-appropriate education about sexual practices. Be clear about sexually transmitted infections (STIs) prevention, and available vaccinations, such as HPV, which can reduce the risk of certain cancers.
- **Risk Assessment**: Be aware that LGBTQIA+ youth may face increased risks for substance use and self-harm. Screen for these risk factors and discuss strategies for coping with peer pressure, social acceptance, and stress. Early intervention and support are vital for addressing potential high-risk behaviors.

4. Fostering Parental and Family Support

- **Educate and Include Parents/Guardians**: When appropriate, provide guidance to parents who support their child's emotional well-being. Parents who may be unfamiliar with LGBTQIA+ issues can benefit from information that helps them better understand the crucial need for parental support.
- **Navigating Disclosure**: For youth who may not be "out" to their families, it's crucial to respect their boundaries and let them guide the conversation regarding family disclosure. Offer resources for parents and families to build understanding, such as support groups or literature on LGBTQIA+ youth health.

5. Connecting with Community Resources

- **Referrals to LGBTQIA+ Resources**: Familiarize yourself with local LGBTQIA+ youth organizations, behavioral health providers, and support groups. These resources can provide community, peer support, and further assistance, reinforcing the care provided in the clinical setting.
- **Empowerment through Advocacy**: Encourage youth to connect with positive influences and advocacy groups that promote self-acceptance and resilience. Having a community can be a significant protective factor against feelings of isolation.

6. Continual Provider Education

- **Ongoing Training**: Providers and clinic staff should receive regular training on LGBTQIA+ health issues, cultural competency, and updated best practices. This helps maintain a supportive, informed approach to care and keeps the team aware of evolving health needs or challenges specific to LGBTQIA+ youth.

By following these best practices, healthcare providers can make well-child visits a positive, supportive experience for LGBTQIA+ pediatric patients. Building a foundation of trust can make a meaningful difference in the health and well-being of LGBTQIA+ youth, fostering resilience that supports their journey toward adulthood.

ADOLESCENT PATIENTS WITHOUT PARENTS

Adolescent pediatric patient comes to a visit without parent

When an adolescent pediatric patient comes to a well-child/sick visit without a parent, providers have a unique opportunity to connect directly with the young person and support their growing independence. Best practices for this type of visit prioritize confidentiality, trust, and empowerment, ensuring the adolescent feels comfortable discussing health concerns while respecting their autonomy. Here are some best practices:

1. Establish a Supportive Environment

- **Warm, Welcoming Tone**: Adolescents may feel nervous coming alone, so a friendly, respectful greeting can help put them at ease. Showing a genuine interest in them as an individual can foster openness and trust.
- **Set Boundaries and Expectations**: Begin by explaining the structure of the visit, the importance

of confidentiality, and the role of healthcare in supporting their independence and well-being.

2. Emphasize Confidentiality

- **Discuss Privacy Clearly**: Assure the patient that their visit is confidential and explain which information may be shared with parents or guardians and which will remain private, in accordance with state laws. Emphasize that they can speak openly without fear of information being disclosed unnecessarily.
- **Address Sensitive Topics Confidentially**: Adolescents may have questions about behavioral health, sexual health, or other personal topics but may hesitate if they feel the information will reach their parents. Clear communication about confidentiality policies helps create a safe space for discussing these concerns.

3. Use Open-Ended, Non-Judgmental Questions

- **Encourage Self-Expression**: Adolescents often face complex social, emotional, and physical changes. Using open-ended questions allows them to share more freely about their life experiences, health concerns, and any challenges they may face.
- **Non-Judgmental Language**: Avoid language that may come across as critical or intrusive. For example, rather than "Do you drink alcohol?" ask, "Can you tell me about any substances you or your friends encounter in school or other settings?" This

helps make the patient feel respected and avoids making assumptions.

4. Comprehensive Health Education

- **Provide Age-Appropriate Education**: Adolescents may lack knowledge on topics like sexual health, nutrition, behavioral health, and substance use. Tailor educational content to their age, maturity level, and knowledge, empowering them to make informed decisions.
- **Encourage Questions**: Invite questions on any health topic, creating an open forum where they feel safe to ask even "embarrassing" questions. Providing a relaxed, non-judgmental environment for learning about their health can help fill in knowledge gaps and address misconceptions.

5. Screen for Behavioral Health and Social Support

- **Conduct Behavioral Health Assessments**: Adolescents often face pressures and stresses that can impact behavioral health, including anxiety, depression, or bullying. Ask questions that explore their emotional state, relationships, and support systems, and discuss strategies to cope with stress and peer pressure.
- **Assess Social Determinants**: Inquire about their school life, friendships, home environment, and any factors that may affect their health or well-being. Understanding their social context helps tailor recommendations and resources to their situation.

6. Address Sensitive Topics Thoughtfully

- **Sexual Health**: For adolescents, it is crucial to discuss safe sexual practices, STI prevention, consent, and reproductive health in an age-appropriate manner. This is especially important if the adolescent feels uncomfortable discussing these topics with parents.
- **Substance Use**: Assess for any use of substances such as alcohol, tobacco, and drugs. Educate on the risks of substance use, emphasizing both physical health risks and the legal implications, while fostering a space that encourages honesty without fear of judgment.

7. Empower Decision-Making and Independence

- **Support Autonomy**: Adolescents often seek more independence and want to make their own choices. Encourage them to take an active role in managing their health by discussing topics like medication adherence, setting healthy goals, and understanding medical advice.
- **Encourage Self-Advocacy**: Help them feel empowered to advocate for themselves in healthcare settings and other aspects of their lives. Teach them how to communicate their health needs clearly and effectively and encourage them to speak up when they have concerns or questions.

8. Provide Resources and Follow-Up Options

- **Connect with Resources**: Provide information on community resources that offer support for issues such as behavioral health, reproductive health, substance use, or school pressures. Suggest websites, support groups, and hotlines they can reach out to if needed.
- **Plan for Follow-Up**: Outline the next steps for their health care and invite them to reach out if they have further questions. If appropriate, schedule a follow-up visit to continue the conversation and monitor any ongoing concerns.

9. Document and Communicate with the Patient Responsibly

- **Respect Their Privacy in Documentation**: Document the visit carefully, being mindful of the adolescent's confidentiality. Only include information in records that is relevant and necessary for continued care.
- **Provide Contact Information**: Offer a direct line or a secure way for them to contact the clinic if they need to ask questions or have health concerns after the visit. Knowing they can reach out helps them feel supported and encourages proactive health engagement.

10. Encourage Positive Health Behaviors

- **Promote Healthy Lifestyle Choices**: Educate them on the benefits of nutrition, exercise, adequate sleep, and stress management, framing it as part of their overall well-being. This can empower them to make choices that support both physical and behavioral health.

- **Highlight Long-Term Health Impact**: Explain how their health choices now can influence their future, fostering a sense of responsibility and self-care that supports their development into healthy, independent adults.

An office visit with an adolescent patient, especially one who arrives alone, is a valuable chance to establish a trusting healthcare relationship, provide essential health education, and support the development of healthy independence. By using these best practices, providers can help adolescents feel respected, supported, and empowered to take charge of their health.

FINANCIAL MANAGEMENT

Best Practices for Pediatric Financial Management

Introduction

Effective financial management is crucial for the success and sustainability of pediatric practices. With the unique dynamics of pediatrics, including fluctuating patient volumes, varied insurance coverages, and the need for specialized care, establishing robust financial strategies is essential. This section will explore best practices in financial management for pediatric practices, encompassing budgeting, revenue cycle management, cost control, and strategic financial planning.

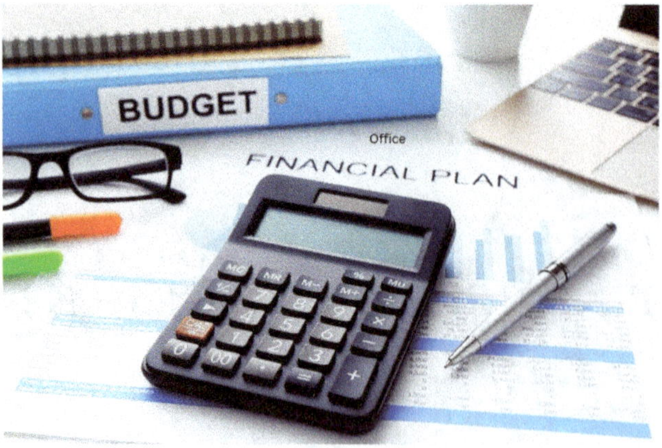

. Budgeting and Financial Planning

1.1 Developing a Comprehensive Budget

Creating a detailed budget is the cornerstone of financial management. A comprehensive budget should include all anticipated expenses and revenue streams.

- **Revenue Projections**: Estimate patient volumes based on historical data, seasonality (considering school schedules and flu seasons), and potential growth.
- **Expense Estimation**: Include fixed costs (rent, salaries) and variable costs (medical supplies, utilities). Factor in unexpected expenses such as emergency repairs or staffing shortages.

1.2 Regular Financial Reviews

Conduct monthly financial reviews to compare actual performance against the budget. Identify variances and adjust forecasts accordingly.

- **Key Performance Indicators (KPIs)**: Monitor KPIs such as accounts receivable days, profit margins, and patient wait times.
- **Trend Analysis**: Track financial trends to predict future performance and adjust strategies as needed.

2. Revenue Cycle Management

2.1 Optimizing Billing Processes

Efficient billing processes ensure timely payment and reduce the risk of denied claims.

- **Accurate Coding**: Ensure all services are coded accurately to avoid claim denials and maximize reimbursement.
- **Claims Management**: Implement a system for tracking claims from submission to payment, promptly addressing any denials or rejections.

2.2 Enhancing Patient Payment Systems

Facilitating patient payments can improve cash flow and reduce bad debt.

- **Flexible Payment Options**: Offer multiple payment methods, including online payments, to make it easier for patients to pay their bills.
- **Clear Communication**: Provide patients with clear information about their financial responsibilities and any payment plans available.

3. Cost Control and Efficiency

3.1 Streamlining Operations

Efficient operations can significantly reduce costs and improve the patient experience.

- **Workflow Optimization**: Regularly review and optimize workflows to reduce inefficiencies. Use electronic health records (EHRs) to streamline administrative tasks.

- **Inventory Management**: Implement an inventory management system to track medical supplies, reducing waste and ensuring timely reordering

3.2 Negotiating Supplier Contracts

Regularly review and negotiate contracts with suppliers to ensure competitive pricing for medical supplies and services.

- **Bulk Purchasing**: Consider bulk purchasing for commonly used items to secure discounts.
- **Supplier Relationships**: Build strong relationships with suppliers to negotiate better terms and stay informed about new products and savings opportunities.

4. Strategic Financial Planning

4.1 Long-term Financial Goals

Establish clear long-term financial goals for the practice, such as expanding services, opening new locations, or upgrading technology.

- **Capital Investment**: Plan for significant investments by creating a capital budget and exploring financing options.

- **Growth Strategies**: Evaluate potential growth opportunities and their financial implications.

4.2 Risk Management

Identify and mitigate financial risks to protect the practice's stability.

- **Insurance Coverage**: Ensure adequate insurance coverage, including malpractice, property, and liability insurance.
- **Compliance**: Stay current with regulatory requirements to avoid fines and legal issues.

5. Leveraging Technology

5.1 Financial Management Software

Invest in financial management software to automate and streamline accounting tasks.

- **Integrated Systems**: Use integrated systems that combine EHR, billing, and financial management to reduce errors and improve efficiency.
- **Data Analytics**: Utilize data analytics to gain insights into financial performance and inform decision-making.

5.2 Telemedicine and Digital Health

Adopt telemedicine and digital health solutions to expand access to care and create new revenue streams.

- **Virtual Visits**: Offer virtual visits to accommodate patient needs and reduce overhead costs.
- **Remote Monitoring**: Implement remote

monitoring for chronic conditions to enhance patient care and generate additional revenue.

Conclusion

Effective financial management is vital for the success and sustainability of pediatric practices. By implementing best practices in budgeting, revenue cycle management, cost control, and strategic financial planning, pediatric practices can enhance their financial health and continue providing high-quality care to their patients. Leveraging technology and maintaining a proactive approach to financial management will position pediatric practices for long-term success in a dynamic healthcare environment.

BIBLIOGRAPHY

1. "Pediatric Decision-Making Strategies" by Albert J. Pomeranz, Michael D. Cabana, and Stephen Berman

."Nelson Textbook of Pediatrics" by Robert M. Kliegman, Joseph St. Geme, and others

2. "Pediatric Primary Care" by Catherine E. Burns, Beth Richardson, and Margaret Brady
3. "Bright Futures: Guidelines for Health Supervision of Infants, Children, and Adolescents" by American Academy of Pediatrics
4. "Evidence-Based Pediatrics and Child Health" by Virginia A. Moyer, Elizabeth Elliott, and others
5. "Pediatric Nursing: The Critical Components of Nursing Care" by Kathryn Rudd and Diane Kocisko
6. "Clinical Practice Guidelines for Pediatric Care" by The American Academy of Pediatrics
7. Updates | Infection Control | CDC - December 5, 2023

Guidelines for Environmental Infection Control in Health-Care Facilities [April 2023]

8. Cleaning Industry - Overview | Occupational Safety and Health Administration

9. WHO releases the largest global collection of health inequality data
World Health Organization 20 April 2023

10. https://shop.aap.org/pediatric-collections-social-determinants-of-health-part-1- underserved-communities-paperback/

11. AI in healthcare: The future of patient care and health management
March 27, 2024• *By Mayo Clinic Press Editors*

12. Addressing burden of vaccine-preventable diseases
CDC: Quality improvement (QI) programs June 21, 2024

Benefits of Immunization QI Projects | IQIP | CDC

13. 40 Years of Human Experimentation in America: The Tuskegee Study
Ada McVean B.Sc. | 25 Jan 2019 History

14. What Is Integrated Health Care and What Does It Mean for You? | St. Luke's Health
Dr. Syed Raza, Vice President of Medical Operations, St. Luke's Health June 21, 2023

www.ingramcontent.com/pod-product-compliance
Lightning Source LLC
LaVergne TN
LVHW050344210926
848481LV00017B/1453